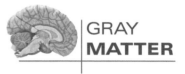

GRAY
**MATTER**

# The Spinal Cord

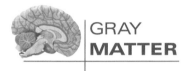

GRAY
**MATTER**

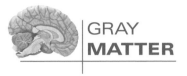

GRAY
MATTER

# The Spinal Cord

## Carl Y. Saab

Assistant Professor—Research
Brown Medical School
Department of Surgery

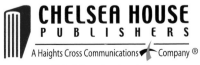

CHELSEA HOUSE
PUBLISHERS
A Haights Cross Communications ✦ Company ®
Philadelphia

## CHELSEA HOUSE PUBLISHERS

VP, NEW PRODUCT DEVELOPMENT  Sally Cheney
DIRECTOR OF PRODUCTION  Kim Shinners
CREATIVE MANAGER  Takeshi Takahashi
MANUFACTURING MANAGER  Diann Grasse
PRODUCTION EDITOR  Noelle Nardone
PHOTO EDITOR  Sarah Bloom

### STAFF FOR THE SPINAL CORD

PROJECT MANAGEMENT  Dovetail Content Solutions
DEVELOPMENTAL EDITOR  Carol Field
PROJECT MANAGER  Pat Mrozek
ART DIRECTOR  Carie Bleistine
SERIES AND COVER DESIGNER  Terry Mallon
LAYOUT  Maryland Composition Company, Inc.

Library of Congress Cataloging-in-Publication Data

Saab, Carl Y.
    The spinal cord / Carl Y. Saab.
    p. cm. -- (Gray matter)
Includes bibliographical references and index.
    ISBN 0-7910-8511-2
1. Spinal cord. I. Title. II. Series.
QP371.S22 2005
612.8'3—dc22                                                     2005011706

*Dedication*
# To all animals sacrificed for biomedical research.

# Contents

# 1 Superman's Legacy: In Memory of Christopher Reeve

## LOOK UP! IN THE SKY! IN A WHEELCHAIR?

Mighty Superman® may fly around and combat villains (at least on television or in comics), but ironically, actor Christopher Reeve—who was widely known for playing Superman's character—a superb athlete in real life, standing at 6 feet, 4 inches high, was confined to a wheelchair for the last seven years of his life, after falling off his horse during an equestrian competition in May 1995 outside Charlottesville, Virginia. Superman became instantly paralyzed after his accident; he was not overcome by kryptonite or a ferocious demon. Instead, his spinal cord was injured high in his neck, and the signals sent by the brain to keep his body alive were instantly cut off. He couldn't move his limbs. He couldn't feel his body. He couldn't breathe on his own. From that moment on, he depended on others as well as an electric wheelchair (which he operated by puffing on a straw) and a respirator to survive.

■ **Learn more about Christopher Reeve** Search the Internet for *Christopher Reeve Foundation*.

Reeve began a fight that challenged both scientists and the public in the field of **spinal cord injury** (SCI) research. In general, nerve cells (**neurons**), those in the spinal cord and the brain, cannot repair themselves. The hope has been that by

1

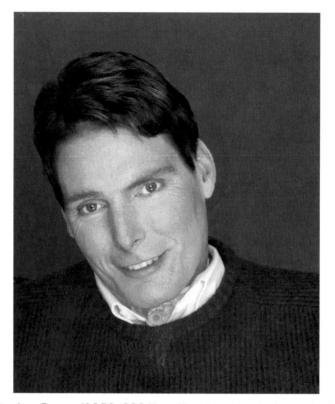

Christopher Reeve (1952–2004) suffered a devastating spinal cord injury in 1995. He spent the rest of his life working as an advocate for people with SCI and encouraging research toward finding a cure.

taking harvested cells from embryos and placing the cells where nerves are injured, they might develop into adult nerve cells and repair damage that the body cannot. Reeve's optimism and determination were resolute: "There'll be a lot of nice years ahead," he said soon after the accident. "The only limits you have are those you put on yourself."

A superb athlete who did his own stunts in films and earned his pilot's license in his early 20s, he twice flew solo across the Atlantic in a small plane. He also flew gliders and was an expert sailor, scuba diver, and skier. Yet, with the simple addition of a thick pair of glasses and a meek voice, Superman® easily turned into the shy and hesitant Clark Kent, often overpowered by Lois Lane. Reeve vowed he would walk again. In 2000, the actor was able to move his index finger, and he maintained a strenuous workout regimen to make his **limbs** stronger. "I was worried that only acting with my voice and my face, I might not be able to communicate effectively enough to tell the story," Reeve commented. "But I was surprised to find that if I really concentrated, and just let the thoughts happen, that they would read on my face."

Courageously, Reeve not only put a human face on SCI but also motivated neuroscientists around the world to conquer the most complex diseases of the brain and **central nervous system** (CNS). Dr. John McDonald, who treated Reeve as director of the Spinal Cord Injury Program at Washington University in St. Louis, Missouri,  called his patient "one of the most intense individuals I've ever met in my life. . . . Before him, there was really no hope. . . . If you had a spinal cord injury like his, there was not much that could be done, but he's changed all that. He's demonstrated that there is hope and that there are things that can be done."

In 1999, Reeve became chairman of the board of the Christopher Reeve Paralysis Foundation (CRPF). CRPF, a national nonprofit organization, supports research to develop effective treatments and a cure for paralysis caused by SCI and other CNS disorders. CRPF also allocates a portion of its resources to grants that improve the quality of life for people with disabilities. "I refuse to allow a disability to determine how I live my life . . . ," Reeve insisted. As vice chairman of the National Organization on Disability (N.O.D.), he worked on quality of life issues for the disabled. In partnership with Senator Jim Jeffords of Vermont, he helped pass the 1999 Work Incentives Improvement Act, which allows people with disabilities to return to work and still receive disability benefits. Reeve served on the board of directors of World T.E.A.M. Sports, a group that organizes and sponsors challenging sporting events for athletes with disabilities; TechHealth, a private company that assists in the relationship between patients and their insurance companies; and LIFE (Leaders in Furthering Education), a charitable organization that supports education and opportunities for the underserved population. Christopher Reeve died on October 10, 2004. He was 52 years old. Throughout his life, however, he was always hopeful, and he stuck to the motto of his foundation: "We must. We can. We will."

Why did SCI confine Superman® to a wheelchair? How can a millimeter's damage to nerve cells in the spinal cord result in irreversible paralysis or sensory dysfunction? In this book, we will explore the mechanisms underlying the sensory and the motor functions of the spinal cord as we look at the basic **anatomy** and **physiology** of the spinal cord.

# 2 | What Is a Spinal Cord and Why Do We Need One?

The answer to the question "Why do we need a spinal cord?" should be obvious to us when we see a man in a wheelchair because of a spinal cord injury (SCI) or a woman who has tremors because of **multiple sclerosis** (a disease of the central nervous system [CNS]). A 1-millimeter knife wound in the spinal cord is enough to cause paralysis of a limb or even an entire side of the body; it could also cause insensitivity to what would normally be a painful pinprick or a gentle touch. Without input from the spinal cord, the brain could never receive information from the body, and subsequently, we would never feel our body or be able to control it. In fact, life without a spinal cord would be intolerable, if not impossible. We need the neurons (Figure 2.1) and their supporting cells in the spinal cord to move, feel, and control our body via intact pathways or communication with neurons in the brain.

## NEUROSCIENCE JARGON AND NOMENCLATURE

To navigate through the nervous system (all of the tissue made up of nerve cells, also called "neurons"), we must first be familiar with several words, most of them Latin in origin: rostral (*rostrum*, or "head"), toward the brain; caudal (*caudus*, or "tail"), away from the brain; dorsal (*dorsum*, or "back"), toward the back of the body; and ventral (*ventralis*,

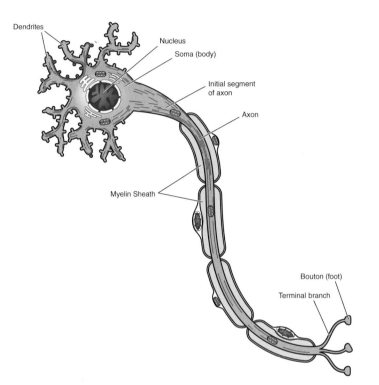

**Figure 2.1** The brain has billions of cells called neurons. Each neuron, like the one shown here, has an axon that transmits information to other cells. The end of the axon, or the terminal branch, typically makes contact with the dendrites on other cells.

or "belly"), toward the front of the body (Figure 2.2). In addition, the nervous system tissue could be cut across different planes to study its **histology**; these cuts can be horizontal (parallel to the ground), coronal (referring to how a crown is placed on the head or "sideways"), or sagittal (perpendicular to the coronal plane in a front-to-back orientation).

Neurons relay information in the form of electrochemical activity via **axons** to other neurons by forming synapses (Figure 2.3). Neurons also require other supporting cells to strengthen the integrity of **synaptic contacts** (discussed later). In each neuron, the machinery for making the proteins the neuron needs

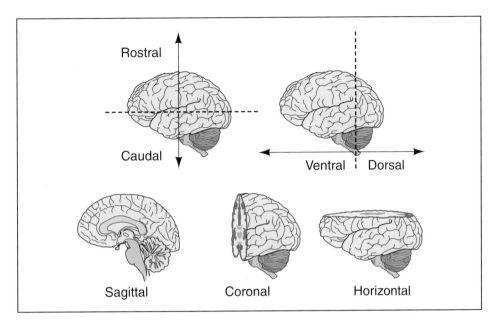

**Figure 2.2** To navigate the nervous system, you must be familiar with these terms: rostral (*rostralis*), meaning toward the brain; caudal (*caudalis* or "tail"), meaning away from the brain; dorsal (*dorsalis* or "back"), meaning toward the back of the body; and ventral (*ventralis* or "belly"), meaning toward the front of the body. Orientation is also described by the terms *horizontal*, meaning parallel to the ground; *coronal* ("sideways"), meaning how a crown is placed on the head and *sagittal*, meaning perpendicular to the coronal plane in a front-to-back orientation.

to survive and function is contained within a cell body. The cell body makes molecules called **neurotransmitters** that are transported down the axon to be released via the synapse, thus affecting the other neuron(s). A densely gathered group of neuronal cell bodies within a clearly delineated space in the nervous system tissue and sharing comparable **morphology** (shape as seen under a microscope) is referred to as a "nucleus." However, depending on the neuronal network within which a nucleus is integrated, nuclei tend to have different functions.

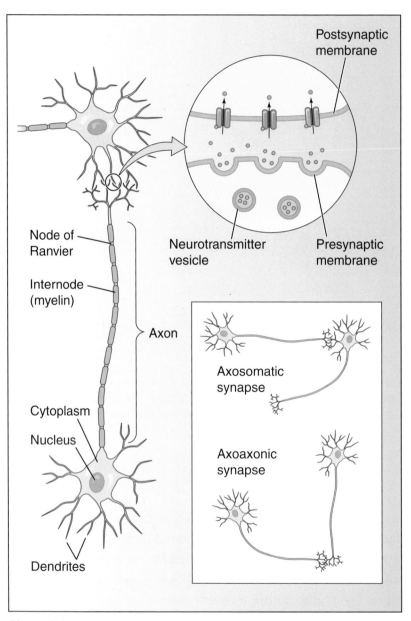

**Figure 2.3** Neurons send signals to other neurons in the form of electrochemical activity. The place where two neurons meet, and the site at which they exchange messages, is called a synapse.

From the cell body originates an extension or the **axon**. Certain neurons, because of how far their axons extend, could well be the longest cells in the body. Some axons may be wrapped in a fatty sheath called "myelin;" this sheath insulates the axon for physical protection and better electrical conduction . (interruptions in myelin insulation along axons are referred to as **nodes of Ranvier**; refer again to Figure 2.3). Dense myelin appears white (because it's fatty), whereas neuronal cell bodies have a grayish color. Therefore, what scientists refer to as "white matter" is made up of bundles of axons—an example would be the outside of the spinal cord. Gray matter, on the other hand, refers to cell bodies (for example, a nucleus within the brain or the spinal cord). If the axon terminal of a neuron is disconnected from its cell body, such as after SCI or amputation of a limb, the distal (away from the point of connection) part of the neuron (its axon and synaptic terminal) will **degenerate**, whereas its cell body may still survive and even **regenerate**; this is the process of Wallerian degeneration first described in 1952 by Augustus Volney Waller (an English neurophysiologist who first characterized this process. (See "Augustus Volney Waller" box.)

---

■ **Learn more about Augustus Waller** Search the Internet for *Augustus Volney Waller* or *Wallerian degeneration*.

The spinal cord is not made up only of neurons; it also contains other cells that support the neurons, such as **glia** and blood vessels that supply nutrients and maintain **homeostasis**. At first, glia were thought to be cells that simply "glued" the nervous tissue together. That is, scientists thought they served a strictly structural role. It wasn't until the early 1980s that more and more attention was paid to the functional role that glia played both in the maintenance of neuronal homeostasis and during **inflammation**.

## ANATOMY: THE SPINAL CORD CONTAINS MORE THAN JUST NEURONS

Although neurons have been the primary target of clinical intervention to combat neurological diseases, other cells, mainly glia, in the nervous system play prominent roles in supporting neurons. Glia in the CNS mostly refer to microglia and astrocytes. These two different types of cells have different origins, but share certain similar functions related to the defense of the nervous system against foreign **antigens** (for example, bacteria

## Augustus Volney Waller

**Augustus Volney Waller was born in England in 1816 and grew up in the south of France, in Nice, until his father died in 1830. At the age of 14, Augustus returned to England to go to school. He lived with Dr. Lacon Lambe and then with William Lambe (1765–1847). William Lambe was a strict vegetarian who thought that almost all diseases were caused by eating an animal diet and drinking the unsanitary water in London. Waller studied medicine at Paris, receiving an M.D. degree in 1840. He is remembered for his groundbreaking work in the study of the structure of the nervous system.**

and viruses). Glia are also known to induce an inflammatory reaction when they encounter an antigen and are activated (discussed in detail later). Once activated, glia recruit more immune cells to the site of injury or infection to help repair body cells and keep the antigen from spreading.

Microglia are derived from the blood, whereas astrocytes are derived from the nervous system itself. Usually, microglia tend to be smaller than astrocytes (hence, perhaps, the prefix "micro"), but that also depends on the active versus the inactive state of these cells. When inactive, a microglial cell typically has long processes ("arms," perhaps to better sense the environment and detect invading antigens), but during inflammation or on encountering an antigen, the microglial cell becomes suddenly more spherical and pulls in its processes, perhaps to move faster toward the zone of injury or infection. Astrocytes ("stars," probably referring to their star-shaped structure with extended processes), conversely, are normally active, contributing to the recycling of neurotransmitters and the maintenance of a favorable pH medium surrounding neurons. When hyperactive, astrocytes also retract their processes and secrete small molecules that trigger an inflammatory response. Some of these molecules are known to act directly against microbes and to attract other cells of the immune system circulating in the bloodstream to the zone of inflammation for **phagocytosis** of cellular debris. Glia (microglia and astrocytes) are therefore considered the resident immune cells of the CNS, serving an important functional role in addition to the structural role traditionally described. The CNS is otherwise impermeable to other immune cells that circulate in our bloodstream, protected by the **blood-brain barrier**. The blood-brain barrier protects the CNS by preventing most molecules from crossing into the brain and the spinal cord, making it privileged territory. Thus, the CNS is immune-privileged, having its own unique defense system, glia. However, it is worth mentioning that the blood-brain barrier also prevents some medications from reaching the CNS to treat CNS diseases; therefore, physicians often have to give local injections directly into the **cerebrospinal fluid** (CSF) through small tubes, called "catheters."

### Inside the Spinal Cord: White and Gray

A noticeable feature of the spinal cord is the white versus the gray matter. If a neuronal tissue is viewed under a microscope without proper histological procedures, for example, fixing and staining, the tissue will appear almost transparent. Therefore, most tissue prepared for microscopy is usually **stained**. Depending on the stain used to visualize the inside of the spinal cord, a zone of darker tissue (gray matter) that is densely packed with cell bodies will appear, surrounded by a "brighter" area composed almost exclusively of axons (white matter). However, it is important to note that this nomenclature may be misleading, especially if a myelin stain is used (myelin is the fatty substance that surrounds axons for protection and electric insulation that actually helps conduction by making it faster and by minimizing the spread of electrical current) since the white matter will appear "darker" than the non-stained gray matter (Figure 2.4). Gray matter inside the white has a typical butterfly appearance, with the tips of the wings resembling horns (dorsal and ventral horns).

### Inside the Spinal Cord: Dorsal and Ventral

Within segments of the spinal cord, neurons are organized according to several criteria. One criterion is the distinction between segmental versus **relay neurons**. The cell bodies and axons of **segmental neurons** are contained within a particular horizontal segment of the spinal cord (Figure 2.5), whereas a relay neuron sends an axon up (rostrally, or toward the brain) or down (caudally, or away from the brain) the spinal cord.

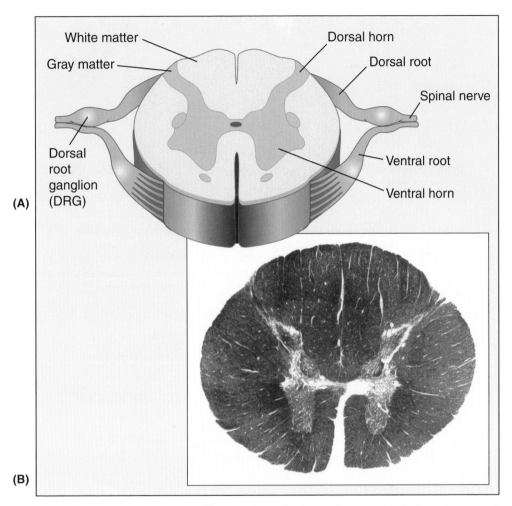

**Figure 2.4 (A)** Staining usually reveals dark tissue (gray matter) densely packed with cell bodies surrounded by a brighter area composed almost exclusively of axons (white matter). **(B)** However, myelin stains white matter darker.

Accordingly, segmental neurons usually synapse on other neurons of the opposite side of the spinal cord or neurons on the same side ventrally (toward the front of the body) or dorsally (toward the back of the body). An example of a segmental neuron is an **interneuron** that may interpose between neurons on

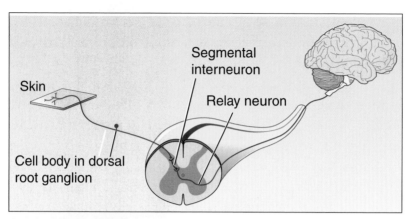

**Figure 2.5** The cell bodies and axons of segmental neurons (for example, interneurons) are contained within a particular horizontal segment of the spinal cord. A relay neuron sends an axon up (rostrally, or toward the brain) or down (caudally, or away from the brain) the spinal cord.

either side of the spinal cord to coordinate alternating movements such as walking.

Relay neurons send information via long axons toward the brain or from the brain caudally; these axons form what are referred to as tracts or pathways, which will be discussed later. Another way to tell different types of neurons apart is to simply look at a spinal cord segment through a microscope and to distinguish between the dorsal and the ventral population of neurons (refer again to Figure 2.4). Briefly, neurons whose cell bodies occupy the dorsal aspect of the spinal cord mainly receive sensory information from peripheral neurons that carry tactile (related to touch), **noxious** (related to nociception or causing pain), vibratory (related to vibration), or visceral (related to internal body organs) sensations. Furthermore, neuronal cell bodies in the dorsal or the ventral horns of the spinal cord form layers referred to as **laminae** numbered one to 10 in roman numerals (I to X) dorsoventrally.

It is important to emphasize here that neurons in the dorsal horn (mostly laminae I–V) relay sensory information from the same side of the body and most send this information to the brain via their axons that travel rostrally in the spinal cord white matter along specific tracts or pathways. Therefore, selective damage to superficial layers of the dorsal horn will result in loss of sensation, mainly pain and touch, from the same side of the body and on that particular corresponding segmental level (understanding this will become even more important when we examine clinical deficits caused by damage to tracts and pathways in Chapter 7).

In the ventral horn of the spinal cord, one can distinguish cell bodies with relatively larger diameter than those located in the dorsal horn. Cell bodies of these ventral horn neurons have axons that exit the spinal cord to synapse mostly on muscles (also referred to in this context as "effectors"). Most of these neurons are therefore called "motor" neurons and relay our conscious (and unconscious) commands to move our limbs. In fact, damage to ventral horns and to motor cells in specific will lead to atrophy (death) of the muscles supplied by neurons exiting from that particular segmental level. This can lead to paralysis of the particular limb, whereas other body parts above and below that level may retain their normal function. **Poliomyelitis** (commonly known as polio) is a disease that affects mainly newborns and children, a drastic example of damage to ventral motor neurons (Figure 2.6). A highly infectious disease caused by a virus, polio invades the nervous system and can cause total paralysis in a matter of hours. The virus enters the body through the mouth and multiplies in the intestine. Initial symptoms are fever, fatigue, headache, vomiting, stiffness in the neck, and pain in the limbs. One in 200 infections leads to irreversible paralysis (usually in the legs). Among those paralyzed, 5% to 10% die when their breathing muscles become immobilized.

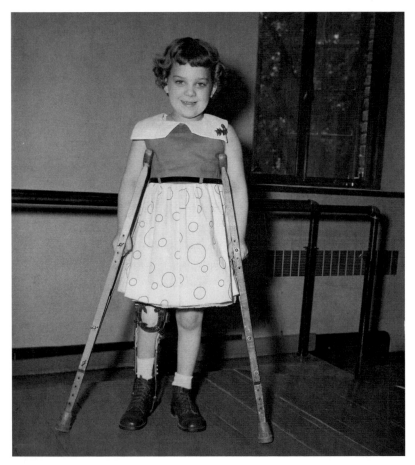

**Figure 2.6** This young girl was a victim of poliomyelitis (commonly known as polio), in the 1950s. The disease, which affects mainly newborns and children, is a drastic example of a disease that severely damages ventral motor neurons.

There is no cure for polio. It can only be prevented. A polio vaccine, given multiple times, can protect a child for life. Fortunately, as a result of a global effort to eradicate the disease, polio cases have decreased by over 99% since 1988.

■ **Learn more about poliomyelitis** Search the Internet for *poliomyelitis* or *polio*.

## The Autonomic Nervous System

Although the term *autonomic nervous system* may imply an independent (**autonomic**) system functioning in isolation from the rest of the nervous system, what follows is intended to draw a clearer and more complete picture of the spinal cord and its functions. What has been presented thus far relates mostly to the ability of the neurons in the peripheral nervous system to communicate to the brain via relay centers and ascending tracts, and vice versa. One distinction is the concept of spinal reflexes mediated by local spinal cord circuitry (sensory and motor neurons) without voluntary commands (hence, these were termed *involuntary motor reflexes*). In addition, recall that most mechanisms underlying sensory phenomena also relate to **somatic** sensory experiences; that is, related to external body organs such as the skin. Within this context, muscles recruited during a voluntary movement can also be referred to as being part of a somatic motor activity, and the muscles are **skeletal** or **striated**. Skeletal muscles are therefore classified as somatic muscles (for example, the biceps or the quadriceps), in contrast to another group of muscles found inside the body, within the **viscera**, called visceral smooth muscles. Smooth muscles are found mostly in internal body organs (for example, throughout the gastrointestinal tract). Almost all skeletal muscles are striated, whereas visceral muscles are overwhelmingly smooth. Cardiac muscles represent one notable distinction; they're found in a visceral organ (the heart) but actually resemble skeletal muscles.

It was also suggested above that reflexes imply an involuntary act. This is particularly true of visceral reflexes controlled by the autonomic nervous system. This system is contained within the brain stem and the spinal cord, and a thorough discussion of spinal functions is therefore incomplete without shedding light on the autonomic nervous system. Though complex, this system can easily be considered as having both a sensory and a motor component, just like the somatic nervous system. The main difference, however, lies in the fact that the autonomic system functions independent of our own will (but not independently from the rest of the nervous system). It controls vital body functions that range from regulating the heartbeat and blood circulation to the digestion of nutrients and production of sweat. In general, the autonomic nervous system handles the maintenance of the body's homeostasis, obviously a vital and complex task.

Imagine that the lights suddenly switch off, and you are left in complete darkness. You hear a hissing noise from an object that seems to be moving toward you with alarming speed. You fall into a state of intense fear. Your heart races, you breathe faster, your blood vessels dilate (you may actually "turn red"), your pupils widen, your mouth becomes dry, and you may even sweat and experience goosebumps (piloerection, or when the hairs on the skin rise up). You're basically getting ready to defend yourself against an unknown and unexpected danger in a potentially serious fight. All of these reflexes occur involuntarily, rapidly, and without prior learning. They also happen almost simultaneously and in coordination. It is logical to assume, then, that they are all controlled by one system, which is actually the autonomic nervous system. In fact, this is all part of one division of the autonomic nervous system, which governs similar stressful situations, also called "fight-or-flight." This division is the **sympathetic** autonomic nervous system. In addition to situations involving fear, this system is also activated during combat, serious competition, or severe injury that results in blood loss. The chief center controlling the whole autonomic system is a relatively small nucleus in the brain, the **hypothalamus**. Other nuclei that mediate commands to visceral organs are located in the brain stem and the spinal cord. To describe the autonomic tracts and nuclei accurately is complex, but it is sufficient for our purposes to say that the distinction between the sensory and the motor autonomic parts are not as evident in the autonomic nervous system as in the somatic system. One way to illustrate the importance of the sympathetic nervous system is the extreme example in which this system is deliberately blocked in an animal within a laboratory setting. Unless sheltered, kept warm, and protected from stressful events, the animal will face serious life-threatening conditions. Conversely, equally important is the **parasympathetic nervous system** that controls basal visceral activity and is recruited during digestion and rest. Therefore, the parasympathetic system is thought to handle states in which one is ready to "rest and digest." Although it is useful to think of parasympathetic functions (for example, slowing down the heartbeat) as opposite to those of the sympathetic (speeding up the heartbeat), or that one acts as the brakes in a car while the other functions as the gas pedal, these two divisions of the autonomic nervous system are not always mirror images. For example, our ability to release sweat from sweat glands located below our skin surface (to keep it moist or for cooling our bodies when it is hot) is controlled by the sympathetic nervous system only. The parasympathetic system has no control at all over our ability to sweat. Most visceral organs other than sweat glands, however, do have dual innervation from both systems.

An additional distinction to point out with regard to the autonomic nervous system is a third division called the **enteric** division regulating digestion and **peristalsis** (movement of nutrients through the gastrointestinal, or GI, tract). This distinction is important because the enteric division lies almost exclusively within the GI tract. Concerned mostly with digestion, the enteric division is atypically somewhat independent of the spinal cord and relies on local gut circuitry of neurons that control secretion of digestive **enzymes**, absorption of nutrients throughout the tract, and motility through coordinated constriction and relaxation of muscle groups all along the digestive tract.

A final cautionary remark concerning this complex system is actually a highlight of what was initially mentioned in the introduction to this section: The autonomic nervous system does not operate in a void; it is not totally independent from the rest of the nervous system. Although the autonomic nervous system may not require our volition, it may still be influenced nonetheless by somatic experiences. After all, most of us may have experienced goosebumps from a gentle touch. Somatic input is therefore capable of triggering, or even in some rare cases modifying, an autonomic response, whether sympathetic, parasympathetic, or enteric.

### Spinal Cord/Brain: Where Do We Draw the Line?

The central nervous system (CNS) includes the spinal cord and the brain. The **peripheral nervous system** refers to all of the other neurons, most of which are located outside of the skull, and the bony structure covering and protecting the spinal cord, the vertebral column (Figure 2.7). No major difference in morphology exists between the spinal cord and the brain, except in gross anatomy. The spinal cord (like the brain) is protected by three layers of tissue called pia mater, arachnoid mater, and dura mater (collectively referred to as **meninges**). The cerebrospinal fluid (CSF) circulates in the subarachnoid space, between the pia and the arachnoid (continuous with the brain CSF) (Figure 2.8). The CSF bathes the CNS and adds more physical protection by "cushioning" impacts. Inside the spinal cord, neurons and axons are arranged in a specific order that could be easily recognized if a cut were made through the spinal cord, properly fixed and preserved, and viewed under a microscope (Figure 2.9).

Most neurons form synaptic contacts with other neurons; as a result, many cell bodies of neurons in the brain project to the lower body via axons traveling in the spinal cord. Also, many

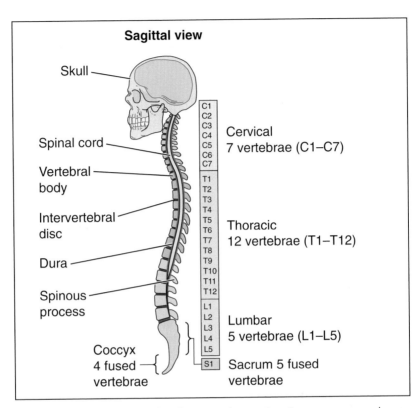

**Sagittal view**

Skull

Spinal cord

Vertebral body

Intervertebral disc

Dura

Spinous process

Coccyx 4 fused vertebrae

Cervical 7 vertebrae (C1–C7)

Thoracic 12 vertebrae (T1–T12)

Lumbar 5 vertebrae (L1–L5)

Sacrum 5 fused vertebrae

**Figure 2.7** The vertebral column, a bony structure, covers and protects the spinal cord. It is divided into numbered regions that are helpful in identifying the site of spinal cord injuries.

cell bodies of neurons located in the spinal cord project to the brain via axons traveling in the spinal cord. Therefore, no distinct line can be drawn between the spinal cord and the brain to separate them into two independent compartments or functional entities. Similarly, the spinal cord cannot be considered completely independent from the peripheral nervous system for comparable reasons. For example, damage to a **radial nerve** that supplies the hand may affect neurons in the **cervical level** of the spinal cord (the portion of the spinal cord spanning

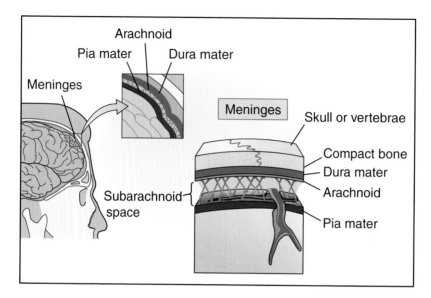

**Figure 2.8** The meninges are made up of three layers of tissue: the pia mater, arachnoid mater, and dura mater. The cerebrospinal fluid (CSF) circulates between the pia and arachnoid mater in the sub-arachnoid space.

seven segments of the vertebral column corresponding to the neck level) by causing exaggerated neuronal activity. However, for the purpose of simplification, the CNS refers to the brain, brain stem, and spinal cord, with the rostral line between the spinal cord and the brain in the lower **medulla** (discrete nuclei located in the brain stem between the brain and the spinal cord).

## PHYSIOLOGY: CONSCIOUS OR WILLED MOVEMENTS
We often feel motivated to "get out there and achieve," which surely assumes that we are able to move, whether that means we are going out for a simple walk or following an intricate plan of offense on a soccer field. No matter how elaborate our thoughts are about how to "get there," we can't get anywhere without

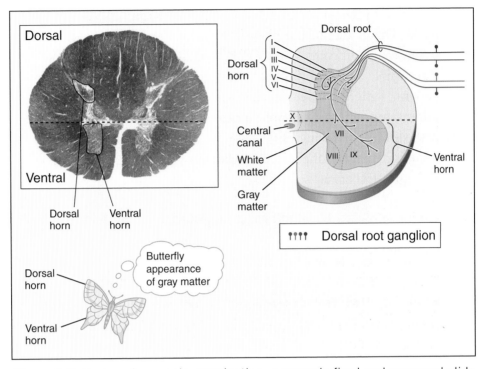

**Figure 2.9** Under microscopic examination, a properly fixed and preserved slide of tissue taken from a cross-section of the spinal cord reveals neuronal cell bodies and axons.

communicating our thoughts to our body so that we can walk, run, sit, dance, or play music. Commands must be sent from our brains down to our arms, legs, and trunk—and these commands are sent through the spinal cord. Discrete **pathways**, a group of axons traveling along within the spinal cord, originate from the brain and travel down the spinal cord to the level of the **effector muscle** in the organ we want to move, with a certain velocity, in a certain direction, and with a certain purpose in mind. This is a voluntary movement. Observe your right hand as you bring it slowly close to your face, then wave your palm left and right. The left (opposite) side of your brain controlled your willed movement in both directions, but the right (same) side of your spinal cord relayed that information to your right hand. This is due to the phenomenon of the crossing over of pathways at different levels of the spinal cord. Knowledge of these spinal cord pathways helps in the preliminary diagnosis of patients with SCI based on the side of motor dysfunction and other symptoms; for example, a **neurologist** examining a patient with difficulty moving her/his right arm will first suspect that there is damage to the left (**contralateral**) side of the brain or to the right (**ipsilateral**) side of the spinal cord.

### Unconscious or Unwilled Movements

We trip on a wire while walking and we almost immediately adjust our **gait** to avoid falling, almost without having to think about it, unconsciously. Once we look back to see what we tripped over, we then understand the event, and only then do we realize it was a wire. Such quick reactions involve an immediate response with minimal or no brain commands. In cases like this, the spinal cord takes over in a process known as a **spinal reflex**. Usually, spinal reflexes serve to protect the body against harmful or painful events that, if sustained and left unchecked for longer than a few milliseconds (the time for the brain to process the information, formulate a plan of action, and then communicate a well-planned response down the spinal cord), may cause serious and irreversible damage. A typical example is the immediate and unconscious withdrawal of your hand from a flame.

Therefore, spinal reflexes help prevent bodily injuries. Although these reflexes are fast and protective, they lack agility and accuracy. In addition, the spinal cord can also take over to a certain extent to help the brain carry out multiple tasks at the same time. Watch a person talking on a cellular telephone while walking around and gesturing. The person seems unlikely to care about the exact placement of his or her feet and the contraction of single muscle groups while keeping busy with mental processes such as arguing with a friend. In this situation, and even in less demanding tasks like peacefully strolling beside a river, we often leave the intricate details of movement (coordination of the appropriate groups of **agonist** and **antagonist** muscles) to the spinal cord, while the brain is busy determining the general plan, such as direction and speed of movement.

## Unconscious Autonomic Functions

In addition to unconscious movements, the regulation of internal body functions is mostly autonomic; that is, they do not require our conscious intervention. Sometimes, intervention is not possible even if we will it, as we discussed earlier. For example, it is almost impossible to willingly control your bowels or the way your heart functions. Although experiencing adverse emotional reactions or anxiety may often affect **gut motility** (how fast food moves through the GI tract), and heart rate may be slowed through meditation and relaxation, these situations are still very different from the voluntary and more precise control we have over our arm and leg movements.

These functions of internal body organs or viscera are referred to as autonomic, and many of these functions are carried out by the spinal cord, so that brain intervention is not constantly required. However, it is obvious that the brain can ultimately affect autonomic functions—for example, by secreting hormones from the hypothalamus directly into the bloodstream.

## Sensations Inside-out

That seemingly trivial question one asks of virtually anyone we meet, "How are you?" can be answered based only on the fact that our body is able to communicate with our brain, the seat of our mind. In other words, we know how we "are" simply because we are constantly receiving information about our environment in the form of neuronal input from our peripheral nervous system and sensory organs. This information travels through the spinal cord to the brain (some sensory organs located in the head such as hair cells in the ear and retinal ganglion cells in the eye project to the brain evidently without need of spinal cord mediation). Even without an overt stimulation from the outside world, our body continuously monitors our joint and limb positions and the state of contraction of our muscles. In addition, even the most common sensory phenomena, such as warmth or a caress, almost invariably affect our mood and mental state. Within this context, it is worth mentioning the positive health effects and stress reduction reported after swimming within close proximity to dolphins and even by gently touching these smart and peaceful creatures.

A set of sensory information from the skin is referred to as somatic, pertaining to the *soma*, or the body, whereas another set is referred to as visceral, related to internal organs such as the stomach or the esophagus. In general, somatic sensations can be pleasant (like a gentle touch) or unpleasant (like pain), keeping us aware of external stimuli as they affect our first line of defense—the skin. Visceral sensations (internal) tend to be mostly unpleasant, vague, and poorly localized when they occur (for example, nausea). We rarely feel our stomach unless it hurts or feels "uncomfortable." The spinal cord conveys both types of information (somatic and visceral) to the brain via distinct pathways.

Ultimately, there is no guarantee that we will perceive a stimulus even if sensory information reaches our brain. Whether we pick up on a stimulus depends on the circumstances related to the event. For example, a soldier in battle may suffer a serious wound yet not realize it unless bleeding is obvious. This may be due in part to the secretion of molecules in the blood during states of extreme stress. Conversely, after admission to the hospital and away from the battleground, the same soldier may shout in pain from the prick of a needle. This anecdote illustrates the capacity of the brain to "judge" the relevance of sensory events before translating neuronal input into perceptions. Exactly now neuronal signals are transformed into human sensations is still a mystery.

## THE SPINAL CORD IN HEALTH AND DISEASE

Neurons in the spinal cord that receive information from peripheral sensory nerves may be connected to other neurons in the brain that, when activated, underlie our conscious sensations and feelings. The specific axons traveling rostrally or caudally in the spinal cord form pathways that will be discussed next in separate chapters under normal or **pathological** conditions.

# 3 | Spinal Cord Traffic

**I was caught in traffic when** the car in front of me slowed down until it ultimately refused to move at all and the highway was suddenly blocked. Apparently, there's an unfortunate car accident ahead! As I reminisce, I start comparing these cars on the highway to individual electrical signals traveling down the axons. The accident suddenly appeared to me like a spinal cord injury (SCI) preventing my car from reaching my final destination. Studying neuronal traffic and highways is, in fact, central to neurological diagnosis.

Looking at a cross-section of the spinal cord through a microscope, one can easily distinguish gray matter from white matter. As discussed before, gray matter contains mainly the cell bodies of neurons, whereas axons make up the white matter. Depending on the stain used, dyes traditionally used to visualize the white matter actually stain the myelin surrounding axons. This myelin provides protection and insulation to neurons, thus contributing to a higher speed of conduction compared with nonmyelinated neurons. When axons are grouped in parallel in the peripheral nervous system, they can be referred to as a nerve. When axons are grouped in parallel in the central nervous system (CNS) (mainly in the spinal cord), they are referred to as a tract or a pathway that forms a highway of communication, sometimes serving specific functions such as pain, touch, or execution of willed movement.

## ASCENDING TRACT FOR TOUCH

Often, the function of a brain region, a nerve, or a tract is deduced from the clinical deficit(s) related to damage to that specific region of the brain, spinal cord, or peripheral nerve. Accordingly, damage to the dorsal aspect of the spinal cord has been linked to sensory abnormality, including the loss of tactile (related to touch) sensation. As discussed earlier, cell bodies of neurons in the spinal cord gray matter that receive synapses from a sensory peripheral nerve are mainly located in the dorsal superficial layers (laminae), roughly around the same segment or entry level of that particular peripheral nerve. Therefore, it could be argued that the sensory loss observed— following damage to the dorsal aspect of the spinal cord (for example, after knife wound) may be due to damage to "sensory" cell bodies.

However, in many cases, imaging of the spinal cord or **post-mortem anatomical examination** may reveal that the gray matter is indeed spared, despite obvious sensory deficit(s). Recall that peripheral nerves relay their pain signals indirectly via axons that travel for a relatively long distance in the spinal cord before synapsing on neurons in the brain for pain perception. It is essential for these spinal cord axons to remain intact for a message to get through, and ultimately, for pain perception to occur. Hence, sensory deficits following damage to the dorsal spinal cord may be due in part to the interruption of axonal signaling and the relay of information from sensory cell bodies in the dorsal horn gray matter. Alternatively, because axons travel in the white matter, a plausible explanation for the sensory deficit would be that a tract carrying sensory information is located in the dorsal white matter of the spinal cord. Elaborate studies have identified that these axons are grouped in a tract and ascend first to specific nuclei in the brain stem and in the brain to mediate the perception of touch from the body surface. Further, this tract is specifically located in the medial aspect of the dorsal white matter of the spinal cord.

## ASCENDING TRACT FOR PAIN

An ascending tract for pain has also been identified (Figure 3.1), located ventrally toward the lateral aspect of the spinal cord white matter. Interruption of this tract, as in the case of injury to the ascending tract for touch, leads to the loss of painful sensation, mainly sharp mechanical pain (pinprick) and thermal pain (touching an object at high temperature, like the surface of a kitchen stove).

   As with the tract for touch, the tract for pain also ascends in the spinal cord to carry information indirectly to the brain (first to neurons in a brain nucleus called the "thalamus"). However, unlike the tract for touch, the one for pain carries information from the opposite (contralateral) side of the body. Although there is a lot of "crossing over" of tracts in the spinal tract, the reader should not be confused about one of the most fundamental concepts of neuroscience: The cerebral cortex controls motor behavior and receives sensory information from the opposite side of the body. Consequently, even if the tract for touch travels ipsilaterally to its input from the periphery, it ultimately will "cross over" again before reaching the contralateral cerebral cortex, thus obeying this rule. Consider the following examples:

1. Damage to the ascending tract for pain on the right side at the level of the cervical vertebral segment (corresponding

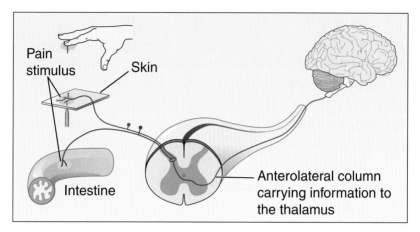

**Figure 3.1** Ascending tracts in the spinal cord mediate sensory perception of both touch and pain. In this example, the tract for somatic and visceral pain is shown. (Another specific tract exists for visceral pain as well.)

roughly to the neck region) leads to a loss of pain on the entire left side of the body up to the neck (that is, pain sensation from the head is spared because axons and cell bodies of neurons carrying this sensation are located above the level of damage).

2. Damage to the spinal cord tract for touch leads to the loss of touch sensation from the body all the way below the level of the damaged spinal segment, but on the same side of the damaged tract.

It could be argued, therefore, that a careful neurological exam does not necessarily require complicated and expensive imaging techniques for a general diagnosis of patients if simple principles such as tracts and their functions are clearly understood. In fact, before technological advances allowed the use of imaging techniques (for example, magnetic resonance imaging [MRI]), neurologists had only these principles at their disposal to perform a basic and reliable diagnosis to answer even the most complicated questions, such as "This man can feel pain in his left hand and leg but not pain from his right hand; can you guess why?" or "This man cannot feel pain from his right leg and cannot feel gentle touch from his left leg, yet sensation from his upper body is intact; what is a plausible diagnosis?" (Keep in mind that injury to parts of the CNS other than the spinal cord, including the cerebral cortex—for example, following stroke— may also lead to sensory and motor deficits.)

## SWELLINGS ALONG THE SPINAL CORD: DORSAL ROOT GANGLIA

On the outside surface of the spinal cord, swellings can be noticed near the entry zone of nerves into the spinal cord, very close to, and somewhat protected by, the vertebral column. These swellings are normal and contain cell bodies of only sensory neurons, forming part of the peripheral nerves (cell bodies for motor neurons are located inside the spinal cord gray matter in the ventral horn). As a rule, all neurons that make up sensory peripheral nerves (and therefore input through the dorsal aspect of the spinal cord) have their cell bodies in these swellings, which are referred to as ganglia (singular is *ganglion*), or more accurately, **dorsal root ganglia** (DRG) (Figure 3.2). As peripheral sensory nerves input to the spinal cord, they form dorsal roots before entering the spinal cord. Some of them synapse on neurons of the dorsal horn, while others continue on to ascend for a few segments within the spinal cord or all the way toward brain stem nuclei. Accordingly, DRG contain cell bodies of neurons of different sizes (as discussed earlier in regard to different axonal diameter and degree of myelination, reflected as increased "thickness"). Larger cell bodies in the DRG are generally assumed to correspond to larger-diameter axons. Because larger-diameter axons not only conduct signals faster than smaller diameter axons do, but also usually carry touch, vibration, and flutter sensations from the skin, one can

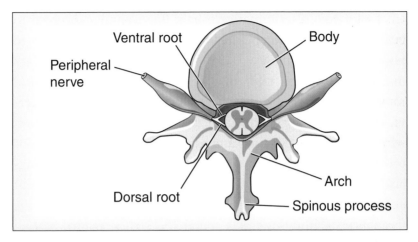

**Figure 3.2** The dorsal root ganglia (DRG) contain cell bodies of sensory peripheral neurons.

assume that damage to larger cell bodies in the DRG leads to a loss of these sensations. Following the same logic, if selective damage to smaller-diameter cell bodies in the DRG could be achieved, this could lead to pain relief, simply because smaller cell bodies in the DRG correspond to smaller-diameter axons that predominantly carry sensations of pain and temperature. This experiment is feasible, at least in animal models, and the results therefore may someday be extended to help many human patients who suffer from chronic debilitating pain that cannot be treated by conventional drug therapy.

## SENSORY DEFICITS MAY ALSO BE INDIRECTLY LINKED TO MOTOR IMPAIRMENT

The dorsal versus the ventral segregation of cell bodies in the spinal cord dorsal horn may imply a separation of function between the sensory and the motor systems. It is necessary to emphasize that, although sensory and motor tracts may well be separated as they ascend or descend in the spinal cord, many clinical cases demonstrate that damage along the sensory tract—for fine discriminative touch, for example—or even in brain stem or brain structures related to this tract can lead to poor motor performance.

Additional support for this argument comes from clinical reports. In humans, a selective lesion targeting the superior cervical level of the dorsal aspect of the spinal cord (at the location where the tract for fine and discriminative touch ascends toward its first relay in the brain stem nuclei) leads to a long-lasting loss of the ability to detect the direction of movement across the skin. It also causes an inability to sense or estimate the frequency of vibrations of a metal rod struck against a solid object and immediately placed on the skin.

Patients may fail to estimate the relative position between two gentle stimuli (for example, gentle stroking with a paintbrush or a cotton tip) placed on the skin, or may even report two closely applied stimuli as one, a test known as the **two-point discrimination** test. Briefly, during a neurological exam, this test measures the minimum distance at which two stimuli are recognized as distinct. At a smaller separation distance, the difference between two stimuli may be blurred and therefore they may be reported as a single continuous sensation equivalent to the distance spanning the points of contact of both stimuli on the skin. Typically, a calibrated compass is used in which the distance between two tips is accurately scaled and visually recorded. Normally, the two-point discrimination threshold varies greatly for different body regions, mostly as a result of the degree of innervation of the skin by underlying sensory receptors connected to peripheral sensory nerve terminals. For example, this threshold is normally minimal on the skin of the hand, and especially on the fingertips where it's about 2 millimeters (more dense innervation of sensory receptors), whereas, on the back (less dense sensory receptor innervation), it may reach 40 millimeters or slightly more. Based on these observations, which rely on a simple and noninvasive neurological exam, significant variations from these estimates could indicate a sensory deficit that may be related to serious damage along the sensory tract in the spinal cord or even in the brain stem and the brain sensory cortex. Accordingly, using this test, reporting a threshold of 4 millimeters or more on the fingertips (a positive sign) generally requires a more thorough clinical examination or even imaging to verify the exact location of the lesion, its extent and ultimately its **etiology** (cause). Most of these deficits generally manifest on the same side of the lesion in case of SCI or the brain stem (but on the opposite side if the injury is in the brain).

In addition to sensory deficits, however, some motor disturbances may ensue. For example, monkeys with lesions similar to those described previously (that is, impinging on the spinal cord dorsal tract for fine and discriminative touch, or on the brain stem and brain structures receiving these signals) exhibit a lack of fine motor control of the fingers, especially evident during grooming, while scratching the skin surface. Furthermore, if these lesions spare other ascending tracts, such as those that carry signals related to painful stimuli, pain and temperature sensations usually remain intact.

Conversely, one of the consequences of an advanced infection with the sexually transmitted disease syphilis is a **syndrome** called *tabes dorsalis*. In this condition, in addition to motor paralysis or severe motor deficit, neurons with a large diameter are destroyed, leading to a degeneration of myelinated fast-conducting fibers in the spinal cord, including those that form the tract for fine touch. As a result, patients suffering from a syphilis infection with *tabes dorsalis* show motor deficits as well as severe deficits in touch (as evident, for example, from a positive sign in the two-point discrimination test), often accompanied by stabbing pain in the trunk and legs.

## PAIN RESEARCH AND CHRONIC PAIN

Pain is defined as an unpleasant sensory and emotional experience associated with actual or potential tissue damage, or described in terms of such damage. But why is pain such an important topic to discuss in detail? More than 4 million people in the United States suffer from chronic neuropathic pain or nerve pain, which makes this medical condition the most costly health problem in America, with estimated annual costs (including direct medical expenses and lost income) that exceed $90 billion. The main reason why most people decide to consult a physician is pain. It is true, however, that pain could be secondary to a vast number of pathological conditions; therefore, pain treatment strategies differ widely. They could range from treating the specific disease that is causing the pain (for example, recommending antiinflammatory therapeutics for the treatment of chronic joint inflammation, **arthritis**) to managing the painful side effects without treating the disease causing it (for example, recommending **analgesics** or painkillers to lessen the pain due to nerve compression by a rapidly growing tumor).

---

■ **Learn more about pain** Search the Internet for *chronic pain* or *pain research*.

Having discussed the spinal cord tract through which neuronal signals relay pain information to the brain, we might assume that one common strategy could be employed to treat all forms of pain, whether it comes from a stomachache, a headache, or a cut in the skin. Mechanisms governing the travel of these signals along specific spinal cord tracts ought to be similar, and hence, ways to interfere with these signals to stop the pain must be common. Clinical practice teaches us a tough lesson, though; some forms of pain are so resilient that even cutting the nerves that carry pain signals does not rid the patient of severe pain. Usually, these forms of **intractable** pain are **chronic**—that is, they develop gradually and last for a prolonged period, even well after the initial tissue injury or disease triggering the pain has healed or subsided. Generally, nerves that carry pain signals in the peripheral nervous system and tracts relaying this information in the spinal cord have been identified and extensively studied, including brain stem and brain structures receiving this input as well. It is thought that this is due to the ability of the nervous system to change and adapt through learning and memory.

The concept that the nervous system, especially the brain, is able to adapt and learn is not new. But in recent years, attention has been given to the concept of learning within the spinal cord as well.

## PAIN WISDOM: A LIFE WITHOUT PAIN?

When the topic of pain relief is addressed, one has to keep in mind the importance of pain sensation. Imagine being unable to detect environmental stimuli that could seriously damage your body (sharp or very hot objects) because of pain insensitivity. This could lead to irreversible damage (such as tissue scarring caused by placing a hand over a hot stove that goes undetected until you smell burning flesh) or even the loss of body parts (such as having a finger crushed in a slamming door without noticing). These accidents are not imaginary; in fact, in a serious genetic defect called **congenital pain insensitivity**, newborns have little if any small-diameter "pain" fibers and therefore are unable to sense pain. This one example emphasizes how pain acts as an alarm system that does not need to be suppressed all the time. Obviously, one needs to feel pain to prevent body damage. It is only when pain indicates a grave or potentially serious medical condition, becomes intolerable, or lasts for months or years (in other words, no longer serves a "beneficial" function) that one should seek medical advice and treatment. The wisdom of using medication to treat all forms of pain, even the milder ones, is therefore debatable. Note that the more painful an event is, the more solid is its memory. Stated differently, perhaps the things we remember most are the things that hurt us most. As a result, pain could be a great teacher. I will never forget to wear the proper shoes for playing basketball instead of a worn-out pair of running shoes, since my severely painful ankle injury after a clumsy rebound could easily have been prevented.

## INFLAMMATION TRIGGERS SPINAL CORD LEARNING

A prerequisite for learning is memory; one cannot expect to learn if one is unable to commit to memory a subject or an act by storing the information (memorization) and retrieving it later on demand (recalling stored information; remembering). Based on the time between memorizing and recalling, a memory could be classified as either short-term or long-term. For example, if you've just been reading through this whole chapter, reciting the main idea introduced in the previous paragraph may be a good test of your short-term memory, which surely also depends on your level of commitment to learn, to pay attention to the words, and to focus on the subject (distracted readers, even if reading out loud, would not properly recall what they've just read). An example of long-term memory is the ability to recall who won the last Superbowl or what you wore on your first day of school. It is generally agreed that memory mechanisms lie mostly in the brain. This belief is supported by at least one notorious condition, **Alzheimer's disease**, which causes the death of neurons in the brain and severe memory loss. The spinal cord is also capable of retaining information in the form of molecular changes that could lead to sensory changes as well. Some of these memories are chronic, abnormal, and could lead to chronic pain.

---

■ **Learn more about Alzheimer's disease** Search the Internet for *Alzheimer's disease.*

An **acute** and moderately painful stimulus such as a pinprick is not supposed to have a lasting impact on the sensory system. In other words, as the pinprick disappears, a second similar application is probably going to initiate a pain response comparable with the first in intensity and quality. Conversely, if the skin is severely cut by a sharp object (like if you accidentally slide a kitchen knife over your finger while preparing salad), the wound may take a while to heal, and exposed tissue underneath the skin initiates an inflammatory reaction (a reaction that occurs in the affected cells and adjacent tissues in response to an injury or abnormal stimulation caused by a physical, chemical, or biological substance) that may delay rapid healing. During inflammation, five signs are evident:

1. Redness due to dilation of local blood vessels, presumably to supply the injured area with more immune cells to help defend against invading **pathogens.**
2. Swelling caused by blood fluid leaking out through dilated blood vessels.
3. Heat caused by vascular dilation and increased cellular metabolic activity at the injury site (immune cell reactions and secretion of enzymes and other factors to degrade pathogens).
4. Pain from continuous stimulation of pain nerve fibers by molecules secreted in the inflamed site and impacting on these fiber endings.
5. Loss of function of the affected organ or limb in cases of severe inflammation.

When immune cells invade the inflamed territory, they begin secreting molecules, some of which are referred to as "inflammatory mediators" and help degrade invading bacteria or viruses. In general, even if a sharp object like a kitchen knife penetrates the skin and the cut looks clean, unless it is **sterile**, it will almost certainly harbor microbial pathogens on its surface that will be introduced into the bloodstream through the broken skin. In any case, this reaction or "fight" between pathogens and resident immune cells is accompanied by the presence of inflammatory mediators that could adversely affect neurons in the area. This would cause spontaneous discharge of action potentials from these neurons, thus resulting in pain in the absence of an overt painful stimulus, in addition to an increased pain response to a painful stimulus.

This increased pain response is an important point in understanding spinal cord memory mechanisms. In this case, the previously painful stimulus (knife cut), if applied again, will result in a more intense pain perception. Indeed, a gentle touch to the site of injury could be perceived as pain (hence, one often guards the injured limb as a protective response). This proves that the system underlying pain perception is not rigid. It can change, adapt, and learn. The mechanisms for this learning lie within the cellular and molecular properties of the spinal cord. The typical phenomenon of experiencing a more intense pain in response to an initially painful stimulus is related to the sensitization of the neuronal circuitry that relays pain signals. This could be easily demonstrated, for example, by recording electrical activity from a neuron in the spinal cord dorsal horn at a lumbar level while applying a painful stimulus to the leg ipsilaterally before and after inducing an inflammatory reaction. The response of the same neuron to the same painful stimulus in terms of number or frequency of action potentials generated becomes elevated. The neuron in the spinal cord has learned to respond differently, thanks to molecular cues released from immune cells at the inflammatory site, which then cause these peripheral neurons to release specific neurotransmitters from their central endings within the spinal cord and trigger long-lasting molecular changes in the form of long-term memory.

## DESCENDING TRACT FOR WILLED MOVEMENT

You might be able to guess that an interruption in the descending pathway for willed movement leads to an inability to move a body part at will, referred to as paralysis. The cell bodies of this tract are located in an area of the brain referred to as the motor area in the cerebral cortex. This motor tract travels dorsally in the lateral aspect of the spinal cord white matter. Damage to the right motor area of the cerebral cortex leads to paralysis on the left side of the body, whereas damage to the axons of this descending tract in the spinal cord leads to paralysis on the same side of the body. Therefore, it is reasonable to assume that axons of this descending tract cross at the level of the brain stem from the right to the left side and vice versa, before finally synapsing on spinal cord neurons that project to effector muscles (muscles attached to joints or bones to allow purposeful movement). In addition, selective damage to the axons that form the descending tract alone, while sparing cell bodies in the brain motor area, leads to paralysis only below the level of damage; for example, SCI at the level of the upper back may result in paralysis of the legs while the upper body and arms are spared.

## ENLARGEMENTS IN THE SPINAL CORD

The tracts discussed previously and others form the white matter of the spinal cord surrounding the gray matter. Imagine the large space occupied by our hands and legs, the need to accomplish fine motor movements with our fingers, and the ability to walk or run. All these functions require more neurons than, for example, are needed to relay fine discriminative touch sensation from the back. This doesn't mean that the back of the body is less important than the hands, but the skills we need to survive (such as making proper tools to forage, hunt, and prepare food, from an evolutionary point of view) rely more heavily on the limbs than on other external body parts. As a result, relatively more neurons are needed to relay motor commands to the hands, arms, legs, and feet and to receive valuable sensory information from these organs. After all, to guess the temperature or the material of an object, it is more common to touch it with our hands—not our back!

It is also true that the fingertips are more sensitive than the skin surface of the back or the belly, because more neurons supply our skin on the hands. Now imagine all these sensory neurons traveling together in nerve bundles a relatively long distance in the arm from the hand toward the spinal cord. Those that synapse on cell bodies of neurons in the gray matter dorsal superficial horn form ascending sensory tracts. Because these tracts carry sensory information from the hand, they will make up thicker tracts as they form at the cervical spinal level (the level at which nerves from the hand input to the spinal cord). Actually, the outside of the spinal cord at this level also looks thicker, even without a microscope. This region in the upper part of the spinal cord is called the "cervical enlargement" (Figure 3.3). This enlargement is partly due to motor nerves supplying the hands to relay motor commands for voluntary movement. For similar reasons, a lumbar enlargement exists at a lower level of the spinal cord where axons exiting or entering the spinal cord at that level supply the lower body, including the legs and the feet.

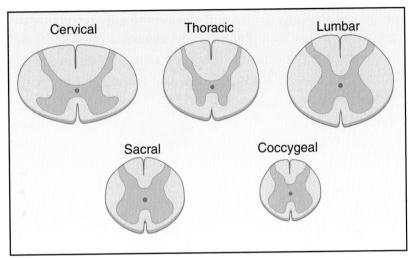

Figure 3.3 Cervical enlargement occurs in the upper part of the spinal cord where tracts that carry sensory information from the hand are thicker at the cervical spinal level.

## PAIN AND TOUCH SIGNALS TRAVEL IN DIFFERENT AXONS AT DIFFERENT VELOCITIES

Not only does touch and pain information travel in discrete and different groups of neurons in peripheral nerves, and along separate tracts in the white matter of the spinal cord, but these signals also travel at different velocities across axons. It has already been emphasized that, in peripheral nerves, myelin increases the conduction velocity of axons. Larger-diameter axons in peripheral nerves carry information related to gentle touch, flutter, and vibration and tend to be myelinated (also referred to as **A-fibers**). Smaller-diameter axons that respond to stimuli that are potentially or actually damaging to the body and tend to be nonmyelinated are referred to as **C-fibers** (although some small portion of thinly myelinated A-fibers may also carry pain signals).

The velocity at which large myelinated A-fibers conduct electrical impulses is roughly 30 to 100 meters per second in humans, whereas C-fibers conduct more slowly, at roughly 0.5 to 1 meter per second. For example, electrical impulses travel 100 times faster along an A-fiber conducting at 100 meters per second than they do along a C-fiber conducting at 1 meter per second. Imagine a scenario in which someone hits her or his elbow hard enough to feel pain. Both A- and C-fibers supplying the elbow region on the skin and deep tissue in the elbow joint will be activated at the same time, but the electrical impulses generated by the mechanical stimulus (physical impact) will travel at different velocities (much faster in A-fibers). Consequently, A-fibers will relay their information to the brain before the C-fibers do. Therefore, the sensation of touch will be perceived before the feeling of pain. Actually, the time lag between touch and pain elicited by the same stimulus could be estimated very roughly by measuring the distance between the point of contact on the elbow and the brain (for example, if this distance is 1 meter, the feeling of touch occurs very roughly 0.01 second after the incident, followed 1 second later by pain). It is imperative to note that this oversimplification may be misleading, because more delays are expected as a result of multiple synapses (to use the example of traffic, this could be compared to more red lights along the way). In addition, once peripheral neurons input to the spinal cord, whether A- or C-fibers, all axons in the spinal cord tract become myelinated and therefore conduct at high velocities. Therefore, the estimated times for occurrence of the sensory perception discussed in the previous example are slightly different than in reality. Sensations might be perceived differently than what was estimated in the example, but the argument regarding the lag between different sensations, though perhaps a bit exaggerated, is still valid.

# 4 Electrophysiology: Neurons in Action

One basic principle of life is change, and neurons help living organisms detect and respond to these changes quickly for adaptation and survival. Although neurons are not the only cells that can respond to environmental changes, they're one of the few types of living cells capable of communicating using electrochemical signals and are hence classified as "excitable" cells because they can produce electricity. **Electric voltage produced by a neuron**, a potential gradient created by charge separation, can be measured. It can also be a reliable indicator of a neuron's state of activity. How can we catch neurons in the act of signal transmission and monitor their state of activity? **Electrophysiology** is the study of neuronal activity using techniques that measure electric current or voltage changes.

## ELECTROPHYSIOLOGY

The physical event in a neuron, its electrochemical activity, is directly linked to its biological activity. In this case, we have a living system, a biological tissue capable of producing physical energy in the form of current, which, if we could directly measure it, can give us valuable insight into its function. Because neurons make up the brain and the spinal cord, this measure may reveal to us the workings of the nervous system, and perhaps even the mind.

Neuronal membranes contain pores referred to as channels that, when open, allow small charged molecules to move across the membrane. Because these small **molecules carry charges**, their motion across the membrane creates a transient current and voltage differential. Although regarded as highly sophisticated, electrophysiology relies on simple basic principles to record these currents or voltages. Individual neurons cannot be seen without a microscope, so it is logical to assume that the miniature current or voltage they produce cannot be recorded by conventional household devices. A sensor needs to be carefully brought close to a neuron to minimize tissue damage, especially in the brain (sometimes the sensor may be placed inside of the neuron as well) and that sensor needs to be connected to an amplifier to boost the neuronal signal. The sensor is generally in the form of a thin needle, referred to as an electrode, or in the case of very thin sensors, a microelectrode, with perhaps the dimensions (diameter) of a hair.

Typical electrodes are made of metal or glass. For metal electrodes, copper or tungsten wires could be used. For glass, capillaries (cylinder shapes of 1- to 2-mm diameter) are stretched under high temperature to yield thin microelectrodes several hundredths of a **micrometer** diameter. Because metal wire electrodes conduct electric current readily (low resistance), whereas those made of glass are nonconductive (very high resistance), glass electrodes can be filled with a solution (conductive), and a metal wire is then inserted inside the glass capillary. Both types of electrodes, with their tips proximal to the neuron, are then connected to an amplifier to boost the neuronal signal. Often, that same signal is also connected to an audio system that allows researchers to "hear" neuronal activity, while that same activity may simultaneously be displayed visually on a screen monitor (similar to monitoring heart activity). Obviously, monitoring brain activity is not trivial, and usually requires recording such activity on a computer for thorough analysis.

## OTHER METHODS OF RECORDING NEURONAL ACTIVITY

Electrophysiology is a "real-time" indicator of neuronal activity using physical techniques (measurement of electric current or, in special cases, voltage changes). Other methods relying on physical techniques that could also be exploited are based on electromagnetic principles, in particular functional magnetic resonance imaging (fMRI). Using fMRI allows the physician first to scan neuronal activity inside the brain or the spinal cord and to localize areas of increased or decreased activity due to trauma or disease. This is based on sensors that, unlike microelectrodes, are noninvasive and detect minimal changes in oxygen or glucose consumption of neuronal tissue. Because oxygen and glucose are continuously being consumed by neurons (in fact, deprivation of glucose and oxygen for more than three minutes may result in neuronal death and, most importantly, irreversible brain damage such as occurs in cases of near-drowning), the scans obtained by fMRI thus reveal areas of high (or low) neuronal consumption of oxygen or glucose, therefore high (or low) activity.

Although widely considered the preferred neurological experimental tools, fMRI scans provide only a rough estimate of neuronal activity within a given area of the central nervous system (CNS). They do not provide a view of individual neuron activity as in electrophysiology. In addition, although they provide marvelous anatomical pictures that are correlated with neuronal activity without surgery, fMRI scans take time to process and show only neuronal activity at individual time points in retrospect, rather than continuous recording (similar to "taking pictures" of an event instead of continuously filming it).

### Examples of Neuronal Recording or Stimulation

The brain and the spinal cord are well protected by bone and strong connective tissue (the skull for the brain and the vertebral

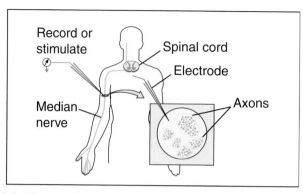

**Figure 4.1** Electrophysiology is one tool neurosurgeons and neurologists use to verify fine anatomical landmarks in the nervous system or to diagnose neurological disorders. This figure illustrates an electrode implanted to stimulate (by passing electric current) or record from the median nerve. (Inset shows location of the tip of the microelectrode near axons within the nerve.)

column for the spinal cord). Gaining access to neurons in the CNS requires invasive techniques (surgery). Therefore, recording neuronal activity is not common in humans for ethical considerations—most often, the benefits do not outweigh the risks. However, in rare cases, neurosurgeons may rely on electrophysiology methods to verify fine anatomical landmarks in the brain or the spinal cord during a high-risk surgery (Figure 4.1).

For example, one treatment for **Parkinson's disease** requires stimulation of specific brain nuclei (basal ganglia) to compensate for the deficiency in a neurotransmitter (dopamine). In addition to the imaging for accurate localization of the electrode, minimal current pulses can also be delivered through the electrode as it travels down the brain to stimulate different brain regions within the vicinity of the electrode tip. Depending on the behavioral reaction of the patient, the exact location of the electrode may then be estimated based on prior knowledge of the anatomy of the brain.

■ **Learn more about Parkinson's disease** Search the Internet for *Parkinson's disease.*

# 5 | Spinal Reflexes

Though mostly involuntary, spinal reflexes (automated involuntary movements) are useful when performing accurate and purposeful voluntary types of movement as well. For example, the desire to move an arm to reach for a book on a desk indeed focuses on the arm while, simultaneously, involuntarily adjusting one's balance along the body's shifting center of gravity through spinal cord reflexes. This resembles the situation in which an army general (the brain) communicates with all combatants (the peripheral nerves and muscles) by passing orders to the commander on the field (the spinal cord) rather than to each soldier individually. The commands do not have to be too specific; they could simply be, for example, "attack" or "retreat," leaving it to the field commander to come up with a detailed plan to carry out the mission, without bothering the general with specific logistic details (fuel, housing, food, etc.).

## COORDINATED PATTERNS OF MOVEMENTS

One familiar example of a spinal reflex discussed previously is the rapid withdrawal of a limb in response to a painful stimulus. On touching the surface of a hot stove with the hand, the same hand is rapidly withdrawn from the stove. This occurs so quickly that the brain does not receive accurate

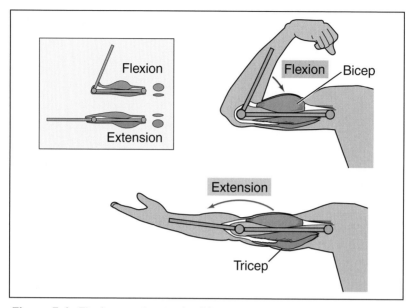

**Figure 5.1** Flexion contracts the bicep muscles so that the forearm lifts. Extension contracts the tricep muscles, which straightens the forearm.

information about the event, and therefore one is not aware of this act until a few hundredths of a second after it happens. Hence, this act of withdrawal following a noxious or painful stimulus is mediated by a spinal reflex. Though basic and simple in appearance, this reflex not only recruits the muscles of the hand, but may also affect muscles of the whole arm, or even the legs. Depending on the intensity and the circumstances of the painful stimulus (in this specific example, the temperature of the stove or the unpredictability of the event), withdrawal of the hand may be accompanied by lifting of the whole arm or even "jumping up" in pain.

Let us consider first the withdrawal of the arm in response to a moderate heat stimulus. Lifting the forearm requires contraction of the biceps muscles (this can be verified by **flexing the forearm** [Figure 5.1] and noticing the biceps contract, feeling "harder"). However, the forearm is certainly also capable of

**stretching** under normal circumstances. This is achieved by contraction of the triceps muscles, which can be similarly verified by extending (stretching) the forearm and feeling the triceps contract in the back of the arm. Normally, both types of muscles (and other types as well) contribute to varying degrees of tension during any movement of the forearm. Each muscle normally contributes in the opposite way. That is, the triceps contract while the biceps relax, and vice versa (however, also refer to **static muscle contraction** as a counterexample). This becomes evident when studying the anatomy of the arm with the insertion of these muscles around the elbow joint; they simply bring about opposite movements when stimulated. Consequently, in a typical withdrawal reflex of the hand (also called a "flexion reflex"), the biceps contract while the triceps relax. These two groups of muscles are therefore referred to as antagonistic.

## SPINAL REFLEXES RECRUIT SPECIFIC SETS OF NEURONS AND MUSCLES

Stepping on a sharp piece of broken glass initiates another similarly coordinated spinal withdrawal reflex—one that causes the entire leg to withdraw. In this case, however, balance needs to be maintained to prevent falling. Therefore, in addition to the activation of antagonistic groups of muscles to lift (flex) the affected leg, another group of muscles is recruited in the other leg to counteract this sudden upset in the balance and mainly produce opposite effects (further stretching the other leg—more accurately referred to as crossed-extension reflex). In these examples, the sensory neurons that detect the stimulus are **sensory afferents** (incoming; toward the spinal cord), whereas neurons supplying the muscle are referred to as **motor efferents** (outgoing; away from the spinal cord).

These two types of neurons synapse in the spinal cord. The simplest spinal reflex recruits only two neurons (sensory afferent and motor efferent) connected by one synapse. Hence, this reflex is called **monosynaptic**. Conversely, a **polysynaptic reflex** mediates more complex behavior, requiring recruitment and coordination of many groups of muscles. This dramatic example of a rapid and seemingly simple behavior reveals basic principles related to ordinary stepping and locomotion. First, spinal reflexes essentially help protect the body rapidly against severe and irreversible damage by external harmful or potentially threatening stimuli. Second, spinal reflexes may recruit few (only two) or many (at the same spinal segmental level or may even span and recruit neurons from different spinal cord segments above and below the level of the noxious sensory input) groups of muscles, forming, in other words, a functional set of neuronal pathways and muscles to achieve movement. Third, these spinal reflexes may occur without obvious brain intervention or even before the brain has enough time to get involved. Fourth, it is essential to note that spinal reflexes, although requiring only neuronal pathways located within the spinal cord (they still occur even if the spinal cord is completely transected from the rest of the central nervous system), are continuously under the influence of the brain and the brain stem (for example, the brain and the brain stem may set the tone of the reflex but not its actual occurrence). As a result, spinal reflex intensities and the extent of recruitment of proper functional sets of muscles and neurons are not only determined by the intensity of the stimulus but are also shaped by experience and will, which are believed to be brain attributes.

## VOLUNTARY MOVEMENTS ALSO RELY ON SPINAL REFLEXES

Spinal reflexes are patterned to serve as "built-in" systems to achieve more purposeful movements with the least amount of brain distraction. For example, it is well established now that stepping or walking first requires the will to step or to walk.

Such functions or desires arise from the brain. This information is then communicated to the peripheral motor nerves through the spinal cord. At the spinal cord level, reflex patterns are similar or identical to the ones described for the withdrawal reflex. These reflex patterns are activated to initiate stepping or walking. It should be emphasized that, even though it appears that only motor commands are needed to achieve movement, no agile stepping could occur without simultaneous sensory feedback from the legs to determine how and if movement is achieved properly. The cerebral **motor cortex** in the brain mediates agile displacement of the body and prevents jerky movements, probably by fine-tuning and coordinating different functional sets of spinal reflexes. For example, following a **brain stroke** in the region of the motor cortex that is responsible for hand movements, paralysis of the hand on the opposite side of the stroke may occur first, but very crude movement may often be restored to the hand with proper physical therapy (**physiotherapy**). Movements may be restored not because the neurons in the motor cortex regenerate, but because surviving neurons close to the region in the brain that suffered the stroke adapt to the new task of commanding the hand and usually take over, using already existing (and intact) spinal reflexes. The recovery is often incomplete, and the hand movements are less supple (perhaps because the "new" neurons in the motor cortex that "took over" the lost neurons' function are not as efficient in controlling and coordinating spinal cord neurons as the damaged ones were).

# 6 Spinal Cord Injury

Trauma—for example, a car accident or a knife wound that affects the spinal cord—may result in loss of sensation or motor functions or both, on one side of the body or both. The degree of disability depends on the extent of the injury and the ascending or descending spinal cord pathways involved. Generally, and rather unfortunately, severe loss of spinal cord function is irreversible; neurons of the central nervous system (CNS) do not regenerate, with notable exceptions relevant to limited regenerative capacity within distinct populations of neurons.

## THE SPINAL CORD IS WELL PROTECTED

Vertebral bones allow restricted movement between segments of the spinal cord (not sideways but rather a few degrees of minimal rotation along a rostro-caudal axis). These vertebrae are also tightly connected to each other by strong connective tissue. The external surface of the spinal cord is also covered with three layers of tissue, as discussed previously (pia, arachnoid, and dura mater). The cerebrospinal fluid (CSF) circulates between two of these layers (arachnoid and pia) in the subarachnoid space. The CSF continuous with the surface of the brain maintains homeostasis (in addition to the nutrients, essentially glucose, provided through blood vessels), but most importantly, physical protection to the CNS. To better illustrate this point, consider the sound that a coin makes when dropped into the bottom of an empty beaker as opposed to when the beaker is filled with water. If this sound can be taken as an indicator of the force of the impact, then it is logical to assume that the water "protects" the bottom of the beaker from the sinking coin and makes the impact smoother. Similarly, the CSF cushions the force of an impact, whether it's an object that penetrates the many lines of defense (skin, muscle, fat, bone, and connective tissue) or just sudden bodily accelerations or decelerations (for example, the kind that occur in a skiing accident).

## KNIFE WOUNDS

Sharp objects are often used during violent assaults. Knives are widely available utensils, within easy reach of adults. A sharp knife even the size of a finger can cut through the many protective layers of the spinal cord. Penetration of 1 millimeter into the spinal cord is deep enough to cause complete paralysis. Other forms of injury resulting from bullets or car accidents involve hard tissue and bone surrounding the spinal cord, thus compounding the injury (Figure 6.1). For example, some knife wounds resemble hypothetical "experimental cases" in which only certain tracts are damaged while others traveling within close proximity are spared. These injuries result in discrete symptoms that could also be mimicked in laboratory experiments using animal subjects (for example, loss of pain but not touch sensation from the same body surface). Such cases typically involve **spinal cord transection** following injury, either partial or complete.

## IN THE EMERGENCY ROOM

On a typical day in an emergency room (ER) in a hospital located within a relatively violent neighborhood, a resident

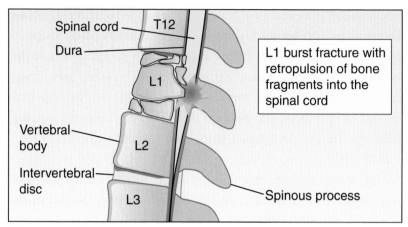

**Figure 6.1** Compression of the spinal cord at the level of the injury. In this illustration, a lumbar vertebra (L1) is fractured and some fragments of the bone, perhaps caused by the force of the blow, protrude backward (dorsally) to cause injury to the spinal cord.

physician may treat a patient admitted on a stretcher, bleeding, with the handle of a knife still sticking out of the back. The physician will probably first worry about stopping the bleeding, if any, and then attend to the damage that such a wound may have caused to internal organs (lungs, liver, kidney, etc.). Assuming that the knife penetrated the vertebral column and lodged in the spinal cord, the first medical response team or the medical doctor will attempt to remove the knife gently in a way that prevents further damage. Certainly, the knife should not be pulled out by twisting or pushing sideways, but rather by withdrawing it along the same penetration track if possible. Next, a neurological exam could be conducted if the patient is conscious. The physician may get useful information from the patient about loss of function using different probing techniques and relying on the patient's verbal statements. However, if the patient is unconscious, the physician may rely on more basic anatomical knowledge to predict the extent of the damage using imaging techniques. If the knife penetrated the body from the back, the dorsal aspect of the spinal cord will likely be damaged. It is obvious from the anatomy of the spinal cord that the ascending tract for touch and vibration travels in the dorsal aspect of the spinal cord white matter, whereas cell bodies of neurons receiving pain and touch information are located in the superficial surface of the dorsal horn. After stabilizing the condition of the patient (stopping the bleeding and repairing damage to organs other than the spinal cord), the medical team will design a treatment strategy for efficient recovery through proper counseling and physical therapy, according to specific guidelines that will be discussed later.

# Spinal Cord Injury in More Detail

Almost 10,000 Americans are affected each year by spinal cord injury (SCI). In 2003, it was estimated that approximately 179,000 people survived their initial SCI. Those who survive SCI go through severe and unique physical, social, and psychological changes throughout their lives, including a decreased ability to exercise. This limitation is especially a cause for concern because most individuals with SCI tend to be relatively young and therefore physically active at the time of injury. A sedentary lifestyle after SCI contributes to a multitude of medical complications, including accelerated aging. However, lack of exercise is obviously not the only concern when considering treatment and rehabilitation options for SCI patients. For a significantly better outcome, a clear diagnosis of the extent of the lesion is necessary for an accurate neurological classification.

## ACCURATE NEUROLOGICAL CLASSIFICATION OF PATIENTS WITH SCI

Why is neurological classification important? There are no standard cures so far for SCI, and treatment strategies differ widely between different neurologists and institutions, especially for different types of SCI. Initial steps toward a satisfactory classification is a detailed description of all the spinal cord dysfunctions associated with the injury. For example, the spinal cord is rarely completely disconnected from the brain except in cases where a bullet penetrates or the skull itself intrudes into the spinal cord due to a very high velocity accident. More often, the cord remains anatomically intact but may suffer **contusion**, **infarction** (neuronal death due to blockage of blood supply, similar to neurological degeneration following brain stroke), or mechanical deformation that interrupts descending or ascending tracts, or even local circuitry. It is estimated that more than half of trauma survivors with SCI will typically have certain spinal cord functions spared and that these spared functions, in addition to the deficits, will give the medical team a great advantage in coming up with a diagnosis and recommending an efficient course or action for adequate treatment.

For accurate and valid neurological assessment, specific criteria have been adopted to systematically examine patients with SCI and to document changes throughout the course of clinical treatments. One system for the classification of SCI symptoms was introduced by the *International Standards for Classification of Spinal Cord Injury*, which was written by the Neurological Standards Committee of the American Spinal Injury Association (ASIS), and later endorsed by the International Spinal Cord Society (ISCoS).

---

■ **Learn more about spinal cord injury** Search the Internet for *International Standards for Classification of Spinal Cord Injury, American Spinal Cord Injury Association,* and *International Spinal Cord Society.*

## PARALYSIS FOLLOWING SCI

The spinal cord generally goes into a state known as spinal shock immediately after SCI, which manifests in sensory and motor deficits, in addition to autonomic disturbances. Incomplete SCI is almost invariably followed by early and late phases of recovery. To begin describing motor deficits, it is important to recall previous topics we have discussed throughout this book. In particular, we need to recall subjects related to the motor versus sensory division of neuronal cell bodies within the spinal cord dorsal and ventral horns and the principal role that cell bodies play in the ventral horn as the final common path to all voluntary motor commands prior to execution. Briefly, some of these cell bodies are relatively bigger in size than the other cell bodies encountered within the spinal cord gray matter. These somatic motor neurons send their axons out of the spinal cord, through ventral roots, and along nerves that travel toward an effector organ, typically a somatic skeletal muscle.

However, exceptions to this rule include ventral horn neurons that target visceral effector organs and therefore belong to the autonomic nervous system. In any event, somatic or visceral motor disturbances may result from SCI. But these disturbances vary widely. Although in most cases of SCI, somatic motor paralysis is evident and voluntary movements in the affected body part cannot be executed, further distinct differences in the manifestation of this paralysis might exist. For example, a **paralyzed** leg may feel rigid to the examiner, an observation clinically described as **spasticity**, with accompanying increase in the tone of somatic reflexes (**hyperreflexia**, for example, an exaggerated knee-jerk reflex) whereas, in other cases, a paralyzed limb could feel soft to the examiner (**flaccidity**) with a reduced size compared with the contralateral spared limb, with absence of evoked somatic reflexes (**areflexia**). These two nonsophisticated and **noninvasive** observations constitute a very helpful diagnostic tool in the neurological classification of SCI. In general, voluntary commands are relayed from the motor cortex in the brain through spinal cord tracts descending toward the motor somatic neurons in the ventral horn. Interruption of this path by injury will result in an inability to move a particular body part at will (paralysis), in addition to spasticity (a phenomenon largely attributed to the failure of the brain to "tame" other descending tracts that mediate this increased muscle tone following SCI). Conversely, if SCI impinges directly on the motor neurons, even when the descending tract for voluntary movement is itself intact, paralysis of the affected body part is inevitable and goes along with muscle wasting (atrophy, death of muscle fibers). There is slight resemblance here between the Wallerian degeneration described earlier and muscle atrophy following the death of a motor neuron. Apparently, if the motor neuron that supplies a group of muscle fibers dies, these muscle fibers will die too. This explains to a large extent not only the flaccid paralysis but also the decrease in size in the overall mass of the body part within which the muscle lies due to wasting. For accurate neurological classification, spastic paralysis generally denotes "upper motor" symptoms (interruption of voluntary commands from reaching the lower somatic motor neurons in the ventral horn of the spinal cord), whereas "lower motor symptoms," mainly due to direct damage to ventral horn motor neurons, include flaccid paralysis and muscular atrophy.

## PLEGIAS

Both types of paralysis discussed previously are clinically referred to as **plegias**. Depending on whether lower extremeties or all extremeties are involved, plegias can be further classified into either parapleglia (latter) or tetraplegia (former). However, plegias could also include sensory deficits as well. These two terms are accurately defined in the following way:

- **Paraplegia**: Impairment or loss of motor and/or senosry function in the thoracic, lumbar, or sacral (but not cervical) segments of the spinal cord due to damage of spinal neuronal elements. Paraplegia results in impairment of function in the trunk, legs, and pelvic organs, whereas arm functioning is spared. It does not include injury to peripheral nerves.

- **Tetrapleglia**: Impairment or loss of motor and/or senosry function in the cervical segments of the spinal cord due to damage of spinal neuronal elements. Tetraplegia results in impairment of function in the arms as well as in the trunk, legs, and pelvic organs. It does not include injury to peripheral nerves.

In addition, impairment of one side of the body is referred to as **hemiplegia**, but this comes more often as a result of brain damage rather than SCI. In reviewing the motor system all along the pathway from the cerebral motor cortex to the spinal cord ventral horn motor neurons, it becomes obvious how a brain stroke on one side of the cerebral motor cortex can cause paralysis on the contralateral side of the body. Depending on the extent of the lesion due to the stroke, both extremities on one side or just one extremity may be involved. In general, however, **prognosis** (prospects for recovery) for motor impairment following brain damage is slightly better than that following SCI. This does not in any way mean than the brain has a better regenerative capacity than the spinal cord; after all, neurons of the CNS do not regenerate (except for a very small population of neurons in the brain that is not related to the adaptive attribute discussed within this context of recovery of function here). It does, however, mean that the neurons in the brain, for example those that specialize in generating motor commands for one extremity, might be able to expand their area of specialization into the surrounding zone of the brain that controls the other extremity, "take over," and generate new commands after physical therapy and rehabilitation. The mechanisms for this take-over are still largely unknown and highly speculative.

# 8 After Spinal Cord Injury: Exercise and the Race for a Cure

$A$s previously mentioned, inability to exercise owing to paralysis is especially a cause for concern because most individuals with spinal cord injury (SCI) tend to be young and physically active at the time of injury. A sedentary lifestyle after SCI and poor physical fitness contribute to a multitude of medical complications, including accelerated aging, a heightened risk of cardiovascular complications (which was the primary cause of death for Christopher Reeve after he battled SCI for years), and dysregulated blood circulation as a result of the malfunction of the autonomic nervous system. However, depending on the level and extent of the injury, patients with SCI can and must exercise for a better health outcome. Those who retain upper body motion can still choose from a wide variety of exercises and sports, whether individual or collective (team sports). We are now getting into the heart of the matter of dealing with SCI, including coping by regular training for building endurance, available methods for rehabilitation, and even scientific topics related to SCI research and the frantic search for cure.

## WHAT DETERMINES THE BEST EXERCISE FOR PATIENTS WITH SCI?

Determinants for a proper exercise program depend on common sense and some basic knowledge of sports medicine.

The recommendations for training to build endurance and strength in persons with SCI do not vary dramatically from the advice offered to the general population. However, it would sound bizarre to recommend cycling for someone with complete leg paralysis, and somewhat more appropriate to encourage a paraplegic patient to take up a wheelchair sport, for example. In addition, special exercises could be grouped into different physiological criteria based on endurance training, resistance training, or electrically stimulated exercises.

When SCI causes upper motor symptoms (reviewed previously), the patient loses volitional control of a particular body limb, but the muscles controlling the movement in that same limb presumably are spared, at least shortly after injury. A good example is the reduced mass of a limb placed in a cast after a bone fracture. When the cast is broken after bone healing, the limb looks pale and feels weak. Even if the neuronal circuitry controlling the limb's movement were intact from the bone fracture itself, loss of function in that limb owing to mechanical hindrance from the cast causes minimal but reversible muscle wasting. A valid counterexample would be to regain muscle strength and mass by physical therapy and proper exercise, or simply by building more muscle mass in an otherwise healthy limb with weightlifting at the local gym.

With upper motor symptoms, therefore, it is possible to artificially stimulate limb movements even if brain motor commands do not reach the intact spinal motor neurons because of interruption of the descending tracts following SCI. In this case, artificial limb movement can be evoked by direct electrical stimulation of the peripheral nerve itself, thus allowing what is known as electrically stimulated exercise, such as leg cycling and leg exercise with upper extremity assistance, lower body rowing, electrically assisted standing, and bipedal ambulation (mimicking stepping). Many electrically stimulated exercises have been approved by the U.S. Food and Drug Administration (FDA), mostly using skin or surface electrodes rather than implanted ones.

---

■ **Learn more about electrically stimulated exercise** Search the Internet for *electrical stimulation and exercise.*

In contrast, lower motor symptoms pose a more serious challenge to patients suffering from SCI or other motor disabilities caused by disease such as poliomyelitis or multiple sclerosis. A multitude of treatments and attempts to reverse the course of lower motor neuron degeneration and subsequent muscle atrophy have so far been unsuccessful. However, the scientific community has learned a tremendous amount about the functioning of the central nervous system (CNS) as a whole in health and in other forms of neurodegenerative diseases to warrant enough optimism and dedication to pursue more research toward a cure for SCI.

Recommending exercise following SCI goes hand-in-hand with recommending clinical counseling and professional monitoring. Because patients with motor deficits are at a higher health risk than normal individuals, especially when they are leading a sedentary lifestyle, they are also predisposed to develop autonomic dysreflexia (dysfunctional reflex of the autonomic nervous system, such as abnormal cardiovascular responses that may result in severe headache, brain stroke, or even death), and fracture or joint dislocation, especially during electrical stimulation. Normally, an intact motor system circuitry will adjust for misaligned, uncoordinated, or exaggerated limb movements. With electrical stimulation, however, limb movement is not necessarily smooth or well executed and, therefore, may possibly compromise the articulating tissue if not professionally supervised.

## PRIORITIES IN SCI THERAPY: STEM CELL RESEARCH AND TRANSPLANT

Immediately after SCI, the injured tissue undergoes many cellular changes and never completely ceases to change for a long period, long after the initial injury, with varying degrees of damage and attempts by the system to repair itself, some of which are abortive, and some of which need external clinical intervention to succeed. Although novel therapies are still being sought, any effective therapeutic strategy will eventually consist of a series of interventions at different pathological stages.

If SCI was the result of a trauma, a direct impact on the tissue by sheer mechanical damage results in sudden cellular death and bleeding. The injury site looks like the messy scene of a cellular war zone with convoluted and rewired nervous tissue and, therefore, interrupted axonal flow and neuronal communication, in addition to local neuronal death, which may cause secondary Wallarian degeneration in other, remote parts of the CNS. Almost invariably, the injury site undergoes an inflammatory reaction. Consequently, immune cells invade the area and initiate a cascade of events for repair and defense against potential antigens. These cells include the resident immune cells of the CNS that are usually present but become activated in severely stressful conditions, including injury. Other immune cells—for example, macrophages, that are usually kept away from the immune-privileged CNS (thanks to a tight barrier, called the blood-brain barrier, around blood vessels supplying CNS tissue)—can suddenly be found at the inflammatory zone, helping in defense and repair, and scavenging cellular debris. However, as in any war zone, collateral damage is expected. In fact, the inflammatory reaction causes significant harm to the nervous system itself, resulting in an expansion of the first injury site to neighboring areas that were initially spared by the injury. To quell this secondary damage by expansion of the lesion due to inflammation, neuroprotective anti-inflammatory agents are usually promptly administrated following injury.

Second, attention shifts toward aiding in the regrowth of axons and the restoration of function. Inflammation also leaves in its wake an abundance of scar tissue, which may hinder the attempts of axons to reconnect through the lesion site. Along these same lines, neurons trying to regrow have special molecular requirements that could also be provided (some of these are called nerve growth factors).

Another novel intervention strategy has focused on the introduction of living cells into the spinal cord to promote repair and, in some cases, alleviate pain associated with SCI. Although focus is on the recovery of motor functions, chronic pain is the primary complaint in a majority of patients with SCI. This is thought to be due to dysfunction in the sensory pathways, similar in principle to the damage in the motor system leading to paralysis. Often, stem cells are the first choice for transplantation (live cells introduced into a host organism; also referred to as grafting). Stem cell biology is one of the most exciting, controversial, and debated fields in science today. Stem cells are gaining ever-increasing favor as a treatment option for SCI. The potential of neural stem cells, embryonic stem cells, and bone marrow cells for reversing SCI symptoms is promising. Put simply, stem cells are undifferentiated cells. They could theoretically turn into any kind of cell or tissue, including smooth muscle, skeletal muscle, the heart muscle, and other cell types such as neurons or liver cells. It has therefore been suggested that transplanted stem cells could replace degenerated neurons if they were genetically engineered for that purpose. Alternatively, these cells could be manipulated to produce and release molecules beneficial for repair, such as nerve growth factors, or even pain-relieving neurotransmitters, such as serotonin, within the transplant site. Advantages include continuous and more efficient delivery of tiny amounts of molecules (growth factors, serotonin, etc.) for a long period, instead of repeated invasive injections with fluctuation in actual drug concentrations within the spinal cord and potential spread to the rest of the CNS (with potential side effects on the brain, which is bathed in the same cerebrospinal fluid).

Sources for stem cells include the developing embryo. However, due to genetic and environmental variations, these populations of cells may have different behavior and responses to stimuli than those of the host organizer.

Finally, it is necessary to retain the advances made by the nervous system to repair by continuous follow-up, accurate update of the neurological classification (through regular neurological examination), exercise, and rehabilitation. Interestingly, even as early as the beginning of the 18th century, Santiago Ramón y Cajal, a Nobel Prize laureate, speculated that to combat SCI we must, "give to the sprouts (re-regenerating axons), by means of adequate alimentation (supply of adequate qrowth factors or protrudes), a vigorous capacity for growth; and, place in front of the disoriented nerve cones and in the thickness of the tracts of the white matter and neuronal foci, specific orienting substances." (See "Santiago Ramón y Cajal" box.)

---

■ **Learn more about Santiago Ramón y Cajal** Search the Internet for *Santiago Ramón y Cajal*.

---

■ **Learn more about Camillo Golgi** Search the Internet for *Camillo Golgi*.

## Santiago Ramón y Cajal

Santiago Ramón y Cajal was born in Aragon, Spain on May 1, 1852. As a boy, he wanted to be an artist. He had a gift, which was later evident in his published works.

At the urging of his father, Ramón y Cajal decided to study medicine and became an assistant to the Faculty of Medicine at Saragossa in 1875.

In 1880, Ramón y Cajal began to publish scientific works. He shared the Nobel Prize in 1906 with Camillo Golgi for their work on the structure of the nervous system.

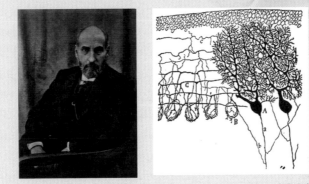

Santiago Ramón y Cajal (*left*) and his drawing (*right*).

# 9 Faces of Spinal Cord Injury and Research

The devastating effects of spinal cord injury (SCI) point to the importance of finding a cure for paralysis and neurodegenerative diseases. The future of research and drug development in this medical field is not gloomy, and the battle to cure paralysis is not over. Physicians learn a great deal from unfortunate accidents and from spending countless hours in the emergency room, treating the victims of stab wounds and motorcycle crashes. Past attempts to treat patients with multiple sclerosis, and the futility of our relentless attempts to rescue them from the confines of wheelchairs, often lead us to admit our own weaknesses and despair. But some who travel this far in the face of tragic human condition also go that extra mile to cross to the positive side, where optimism never fades, where every attempt to trick the disease and improvise new strategies to overcome these great medical riddles becomes a way of life. Surprisingly, patients often express a positive message, which could be brighter than our best expectations. Tragedy is in the face of the beholder! Here is one such story, from my dear friend, Nael Smith (Figure 9.1):

> In 1999, I was involved in a car crash that would bring about many alterations to the way I went about doing things. My spinal cord got severed; this

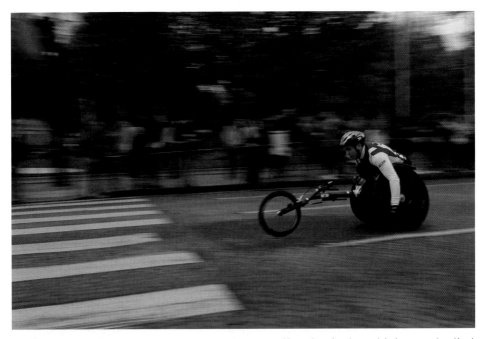

**Figure 9.1** Nael Smith, after a car accident, suffered spinal cord injury and relied on a wheelchair for mobility, but also learned new ways for fast locomotion and athleticism.

meant that I would have to use a wheelchair for mobility. Post–car crash, I realized my body needed to learn new ways of locomotion. Upon its introduction into my room during rehabilitation, the wheelchair gave me immediate mobility and liberty. I was later taught to jump curbs, pop wheelies, and push on different surfaces. I have embraced the wheelchair and do not regard myself as being confined to one; rather I find it to be a liberating tool that gives me the chance of continuing a very active and full life.

Soon after regaining my independence, I needed to find new ways of fulfilling my pre-injury sports junkie thirst. Since many aspects of my life had to adapt, there was no reason that sports would no longer be part of my life. I soon adopted wheelchair basketball in place of basketball, switched from skiing to sit-skiing, and learned how to scuba dive without the use of my lower extremities. Wheelchair racing took on the role of running.

Wheelchair racing has taken center stage in my choice of adaptive (for the disabled) sports. The enthusiasm of developing my skills, trying to beat a personal best, or even surpassing my own expectations, is there just as much an able-bodied athlete. And there is no reason why things should change on that level. Today I continue to train hard as any other sport person would, trying to shave off vital seconds.

Racing has also given me the chance to meet lots of interesting people from different parts of the world. I have come across many fellow disabled athletes who train and work hard in wheelchair racing and whom I can relate. Marathons and track racing meetings bring us together. We would like to, and should only, be regarded as athletes who deserve appreciation because we are hard working and dedicated athletes with a disability. We are not disabled people who happen to be there.

You might be wondering why I race and what it means to me. Is it the sense of accomplishment that keeps my arms pushing? Is it because I fear idleness? A straight and simple answer comes to mind: It just brings me the sensation of being alive. The thrill of punching the rim and pushing closer and closer to the finish line of an intense 26.2 miles gives me that rush that makes me feel life to the fullest. Racing through every borough of last year's New York City marathon had its own share of surprises. The intensity of the cheers of two million spectators along the course made me complete the race despite puncturing three tires!

Racing has affected me and the people around me. The meaning of racing laid in its undeniable power to affect my adaptation to an abrupt new state of physical mobility. I thought I had lost a lot of my physical abilities with the accident. Once I got my first racing chair, the possibilities I grasped were literally endless; it made me gain my confidence back. And this resonated on peers with similar disabilities. Racing and training hard has helped me develop my understanding toward life and what really makes me happy.

---

■ **Learn more about exercise and spinal cord injuries** Search the Internet for *athletics* and *spinal cord injury*.

## ROBOTICS

Traditional rehabilitation training for SCI is usually administered after an acute event, such as trauma, resulting in motor deficits. These traditional methods reinforce individual movement components required for walking, in addition to improving strength and endurance. Rehabilitative patient education has also been traditionally focused on developing behaviors compensating for the deficits. However, in the 1970s, a breakthrough occurred in motor system physiology research when it was announced that a **spinalized cat** (a cat with complete transection of the spinal cord) is able to respond to a treadmill in motion if the cat's body weight is supported. Walking suddenly seemed possible even for patients with severe SCI. Although volitional walking was still out of the question (all descending tracts being severed in the spinalized cat), this research led to the development of a so-called treadmill training rehabilitation exercise with the assistance of physiotherapists. The main hypothesis behind this research was that, based on this experimental evidence, an independent system to generate walking patterns within the spinal cord surely exists. Periodic excitation of the skin, muscle, and joint receptors in the lower limbs evokes input to the reflex neural circuits located within the spinal cord. This system, also currently known as the central pattern generator (CPG), normally produces purposeful movements on receiving supra-spinal orders (from the brain stem and the brain) but could similarly evoke motor patterns if triggered by the sensory input from the lower limbs to the spinal cord (if spared by the injury), thus triggering reflex stepping.

Typically, two physiotherapists move the suspended legs of the patient over an active treadmill to simulate walking. During the training, the body weight of the patient is supported (the patients are obviously not able to maintain their equilibrium and walk by themselves). In a later stage of rehabilitation, depending on the severity of their neurological classification, some patients exhibit a positive outcome and regain the ability to walk by themselves, but they might still require body-weight support to do so. Currently, treadmill training has become an established rehabilitation exercise for patients with locomotor dysfunction due to central nervous system (CNS) diseases such as SCI, stroke, and multiple sclerosis. This technique offers faster and greater mobility improvement, especially when combined with treadmill training and conventional physiotherapy, basically by reactivating the intact CPG, therefore improving the generated muscle activation pattern. The result is a faster and better relearning of locomotion, because the spinal cord is not privy to any brain commands following SCI. Because assisting the patient's leg movement in manual treadmill training is a very strenuous task for the physiotherapists, contributing to limitations in the duration and causing irregularities, recent advances to automate the training system have proved to be quite successful.

Combining clinical and engineering innovations has recently introduced gait-specific training using body-weight supported treadmill (BWST) with robotic assistance. BWST provides the opportunity to shift toward strategies that reinforce the proper activation of neural circuitry controlling gait and activity-dependent compensation. In summary, BWST provides a tool for repetitive cycles of task-specific training. These techniques are primarily intended to rebuild and reinforce the neurological basis of walking. The robotic devices offer an additional level of lower extremity control and support for interactive gait training, which is obviously superior to manually assisted gait-training in terms of duration of exercise, consistency, and accuracy of the desired task-specific movement. These sensitive robotic devices are rather rare and can be found only in a handful of hospitals and rehabilitation centers around the world. One such device is already installed at the Veterans of America Hospital in West Haven, Connecticut. The neurologist and team leader of this research project aimed at functional improvement of motor deficits is Dr. Albert Lo, a young, talented, and tireless assistant professor of neurology at Yale University and the hospital. On September 9, 2004, Lo received the prestigious "Presidential Early Career Award for Scientists and Engineers," the U.S. government's highest honor for outstanding scientists and engineers at the outset of their research careers. Lo acknowledged the award but was quick to note, "achievements are important, but the process and journey of learning is just as important."

■ **Learn more about Dr. Albert Lo's research** Search the Internet for *Dr. Albert Lo.*

# Glossary

**Acute**  Short-term (in contrast to **chronic**).

**A-fibers**  Peripheral neurons of larger and myelinated (A-) diameter carrying signals for fine touch and vibration (A-).

**Agonist**  A group of muscles that counteract another group of muscles, the antagonist.

**Alzheimer's disease**  Progressive brain disorder due to neuronal degeneration that gradually destroys a person's memory and ability to learn, reason, make judgments, communicate, and carry out daily activities. As Alzheimer's disease progresses, individuals may also experience changes in personality and behavior, such as anxiety, suspiciousness, or agitation, as well as delusions or hallucinations.

**Analgesics**  Medications for the treatment of pain.

**Anatomy**  The study of body parts and tissues.

**Antagonist**  One group of muscles that contracts while the other, the agonist, simultaneously relaxes.

**Antigen**  An organism foreign to the body.

**Areflexia**  Absence of reflex.

**Arthritis**  Chronic joint inflammation.

**Autonomic**  Independent, not requiring other intervention.

**Axon**  The part of a neuron extending from the cell body through which electrical signals are transmitted.

**Blood-brain barrier**  Protective layer formed by tight junctions and special blood vessels surrounding the brain and the spinal cord preventing most molecules from crossing into the central nervous system, making it privileged territory.

**Brain stroke**  Sudden interruption of the blood supply to neurons in the brain, typically due to a clot blocking a blood vessel.

**Central nervous system (CNS)**  The brain and spinal cord.

**Cerebrospinal fluid (CSF)**  Liquid that fills the ventricles and spinal cord, carries nutrients, and cushions forces of impact.

**Cervical level**  The spinal cord is divided into several portions spanning the vertebral column; the cervical portion corresponds to seven segments at the neck level.

**C-fibers** Peripheral neurons of smaller unmyelinated (C-) diameter carrying signals for pain.

**Chronic** Long-lasting (in contrast to acute).

**Congenital pain insensitivity** An inability to sense pain due to an identified genetic mutation.

**Contralateral** On the opposite side.

**Contusion** Tissue injury with no laceration.

**Degenerate** To breakdown; die.

**Dorsal root ganglia (DRG)** Cell bodies of sensory peripheral nerves grouped in swellings along the spinal cord.

**Effector muscle** End target of a motor neuron that carries out movement commands.

**Electric voltage produced by a neuron** Difference in voltage between two points (across neuronal membrane) due to accumulation of ions carrying electric charges on either side of an impermeable barrier (neuronal membrane). When the barrier becomes permissive to ions carrying these electric charges (by opening pores across the membrane, otherwise called membrane ion channels), movement of these ions generates current that spreads along the axon creating an "action potential," a unitary electric signal characteristic of individual neurons.

**Electrophysiology** Study of neuronal activity using physical techniques to measure electric current or voltage changes.

**Enteric** Related to the intestines.

**Enzymes** Small molecules that catalyze chemical reactions.

**Etiology** Cause of a disease.

**Flaccidity** Decreased muscle tone.

**Flexing the forearm** Bringing forearm closer to the shoulder by rotating it around the elbow joint upward in an upright standard anatomical position.

**Gait** Posture and slow walk.

**Glia** A diverse collection of cells in the brain and spinal cord involved in maintaining the normal functioning of neurons.

**Gut motility**  The speed at which food moves through the digestive tract.

**Hemiplegia**  Paralysis of one side of the body.

**Histology**  Study of tissues, commonly through the use of special staining (coloration) techniques to view different tissues and cellular components under a microscope.

**Homeostasis**  Stable environment; concept widely used in biology to denote healthy stability in a rather dynamic medium.

**Hyperreflexia**  Exaggerated motor reflex.

**Hypothalamus**  A nucleus, located below the thalamus in the center comparable of the brain, that is the chief regulator of the autonomic nervous system.

**Infarction**  Cellular death due to blockage of blood supply and oxygen, comparable to neuronal degeneration following brain stroke.

**Inflammation**  When the immune system reacts to invading microbes or pathogens, immune cells trigger a cellular reaction or inflammation that could be localized to the site of injury or generalized. Inflammation is associated with mainly five basic signs: redness, swelling, heat, pain, and weakness or loss of function.

**Interneuron**  Neuron that interposes between two other neurons.

**Intractable**  Resistant to treatment.

**Ipsilateral**  On the same side.

**Laminae**  Different layers, for example, superficial layers of the spinal cord.

**Limb**  Appendage, extremity (for example, an arm or leg).

**Medulla**  A group of axons and cell bodies of neurons forming discrete nuclei located in the brain stem (between the brain and the spinal cord). One major function of these neurons is to maintain the breathing reflex. Even minimal damage to this area may result in death.

**Meninges**  Three membranes, called pia, arachnoid, and dura mater, which cover and protect the central nervous system.

**Micrometer**  One micrometer (μm) is one thousandth of a millimeter.

**Molecules carry charges**  Mostly ions with one or two positive or negative charges, for example, sodium [Na$^+$], potassium [K$^+$], calcium [Ca$^{++}$], or chloride [Cl$^-$] ions.

**Monosynaptic**  Containing only one synapse between two neurons.

**Morphology**  Gross features of a tissue, typically visualized with a microscope.

**Motor cortex**  Brain region containing neurons mediating voluntary motor commands; damage to these neurons leads to paralysis of the corresponding body part, mainly contralateral to the brain lesion.

**Motor efferent**  Neuron carrying motor commands away from the spinal cord, mainly supplying the muscle.

**Neurologist**  A medical doctor who specializes in diagnosing and treating diseases of the nervous system.

**Neuron**  The cells of the nervous system involved in transmitting messages from one place to another. A typical neuron has dendrites, a cell body, and an axon.

**Neurotransmitters**  The chemical messengers released by the axon of a neuron.

**Nodes of Ranvier**  Normal gaps between areas of myelination along an axon.

**Noninvasive**  Not requiring surgery or tissue penetration.

**Noxious**  Causing pain or tissue injury or potential harm; for example, a pinprick or burn.

**Paraplegia**  Paralysis in the lower limbs (but not in the upper limbs).

**Parasympathetic nervous system**  Autonomic nervous system division for "rest-and-digest" states.

**Parkinson's disease**  A brain disorder occurring when certain neurons in a part of the brain called the substantia nigra die or become impaired. Normally, these cells produce a chemical known as dopamine that allows smooth, coordinated function of the body's muscles and movement.

**Pathogens**  Organisms causing pathology.

**Pathological**  Referring to a disease state.

**Pathways**  A group of axons traveling along within the spinal cord conveying one function (sensory, motor, or other).

**Peripheral nervous system (PNS)**  Tissue of the nervous system located outside the skull and the vertebral column.

**Peristalsis**  The movement of food or other nutrients through the gastrointestinal (GI) tract.

**Phagocytosis**  Cellular degradation.

**Physiology**  The science of the functioning of living organisms.

**Physiotherapy**  Therapy that uses physical methods such as exercise and massage.

**Plegia**  Paralysis.

**Poliomyelitis**  Viral disease that is uncommon these days, largely because of vaccines administered at early age. In the early to mid-20th century, however, before the vaccine was developed, victims came down with fever and other typical signs of the disease and eventually suffered severe motor deficits or even complete paralysis.

**Polysynaptic**  Containing more than two neurons making multiple synapses.

**Postmortem anatomical examination**  Examination after death, or autopsy.

**Prognosis**  Prospect or expectation for recovery from a disease.

**Radial nerve**  Extends down the humerus bone and divides into one branch that goes to the skin on the back of the hand and another that goes to the underlying extensor muscles.

**Regenerate**  Regrow.

**Relay neurons**  Neurons that relay information rostrally in the spinal cord.

**Segmental neurons**  Neurons contained within a segment of the spinal cord (also referred to as "interneurons").

**Sensory afferent** Neuron carrying sensory signals toward the spinal cord.

**Skeletal** Somatic striated muscles, not visceral or smooth.

**Somatic** Related to the body; referring to body organs other than the viscera.

**Spasticity** Increased muscle tone, rigidity.

**Spinal cord injury** Direct damage to spinal cord tissue typically caused by violent accidents, or indirect damage following the injury owing to interrupted blood supply and severe inflammation.

**Spinal cord transection** Horizontal cut through the spinal cord leading to separation of ascending and descending spinal tracts above and below the lesion. Comparable in many ways but not exactly similar to spinal injury. For example, a severe car accident may result in spinal cord injury *and* transection, whereas transection could further be described as partial (dorsal, ventral, etc.) or complete (complete separation on a rostro-caudal axis).

**Spinal reflex** Involuntary movement mediated only by neurons located in the spinal cord, thus, not requiring brain intervention; usually too rapid to even allow time for brain intervention.

**Spinalized cat** A cat subjected to complete transection of the spinal cord.

**Stained** The spinal cord or brain tissue sectioned very thin and mounted on a glass slide looks transparent under a traditional light microscope without staining cell bodies or axons using one or multiple dyes.

**Static muscle contraction** During static muscle contraction; for example, when carrying a shopping bag, the arm may be stable but definitely tensed owing to contraction of many types of muscles to counteract gravity forces pulling on the bag. In this case, both triceps and biceps may be contracting, each virtually pulling the forearm in opposite direction, with no overall movement.

**Sterile** Free of disease-causing microorganisms.

**Stretching** Extending or moving away from the joint.

**Striated**  Having fibers that run in a parallel direction.

**Sympathetic autonomic nervous system**  Autonomic nervous system division for fight-or-flight responses.

**Syndrome**  A pattern of symptoms indicative of some disease, whereas symptom refers to any sensation or change in bodily function experienced by a patient and associated with a particular disease.

*Tabes dorsalis*  Degeneration of large-diameter axons following syphilitic infection, leading to loss of fine touch accompanied by pain in the trunk and legs.

**Tetraplegia**  Paralysis in the lower and upper limbs.

**Two-point discrimination**  Minimum distance at which two stimuli are resolved as distinct.

**Viscera**  Internal body organs, for example, the digestive system but not the nervous system.

# Bibliography

## BOOKS

Johnston, D., and S. M. Wu. *Foundations of Cellular Neurophysiology,* 2nd ed. Cambridge, MA: MIT Press, 1995.

Kandel, E. R., J. H. Schwartz, and T. M. Jessell. *Principles of Neural Science,* 4th ed. New York: McGraw-Hill, 2000.

Nolte, J., and J. B. Angevine. *The Human Brain.* St. Louis: Mosby, 1995.

Willis, W. D., and R. E. Coggeshall. *Sensory Mechanisms of the Spinal Cord,* 3nd ed. New York: Plenum Press, 2004.

## PERIODICALS

Jacobs, P. L., and M. S. Nash. "Exercise Recommendations for Individuals With Spinal Cord Injury." *Sports Medicine* 34 (2004): 727–751.

Jezernik S., R. Scharer, G. Colombo, and M. Morari. "Adaptive Robotic Rehabilitation of Locomotion: A Clinical Study in Spinally Injured Individuals." *Spinal Cord* 41 (2003): 657–666.

# Further Reading

Kandel, E. R., J. H. Schwartz, and T. M. Jessell. *Principles of Neural Science, 4th Ed.*, McGraw Hill, 2000.

Nolte, J., and J. B. Angevine. *The Human Brain*, Mosby, 1995.

Sanes, D. H., T. A. Reh, and W. A. Harris, eds. *Development of the Nervous System*. New York: Academic Press, 2000.

Taussig, M. *The Nervous System*. New York: Routledge, 1991.

Vikhanski, L. *In Search of the Lost Cord—Solving the Mystery of Spinal Cord Regeneration*. Washington, D.C.: Joseph Henry Press, 2001.

# Websites

Alzheimer's Association
*http://www.alz.org/*

American Spinal Injury Association
*http://www.asia-spinalinjury.org/home/index.html*

BioResearch
*http://bioresearch.ac.uk/*

Brain Explorer
*http://www.brainexplorer.org/brain_atlas/Brainatlas_index.shtml*

Christopher Reeve Foundation
*http://www.christopherreeve.org/*

Cleveland Clinic (on inflammation)
*http://www.clevelandclinic.org/health/health-info/docs/0200/0217.asp?index=4857*

International Association of Pain
*http://www.iasp-pain.org/terms-p.html*

International Spinal Cord Society
*http://www.iscos.org.uk/*

International Standards for Classification of Spinal Cord Injury
*http://www.asia-spinalinjury.org/publications/2001_Classif_work-sheet.pdf*

National Multiple Sclerosis Society
*http://www.nationalmssociety.org/What%20is%20MS.asp*

National Parkinson Foundation
*http://www.parkinson.org/site/pp.asp?c=9dJFJLPwB&b=71117*

Neuroscience for Kids
*http://faculty.washington.edu/chudler/neurok.html*

Nobel Prize
*http://nobelprize.org/index.html*

Nucleus Medical Arts
*http://catalog.nucleusinc.com/catalogindex.php*

The U.S. Food and Drug Administration *http://www.fda.gov/*

Virtual Hospital
*http://www.vh.org/welcome/aboutus/index.html*

WhoNamedIt
*http://www.whonamedit.com/*

WHO on Poliomyelitis
*http://www.who.int/topics/poliomyelitis/en/*

Yale Scientific
*http://research.yale.edu/ysm/index.jsp?issue=78.1*

Yale University, Department of Neurology
*http://info.med.yale.edu/neurol/index.html*

# Index

# About the Author

**Carl Y. Saab** is an active neuroscience researcher. He graduated in 1997 from the American University of Beirut (AUB) in Lebanon with an M.S. in neuroscience. At AUB, he learned the principles of pain research, devoting his time to working closely with Dr. Nayef Saadé at the department of human morphology. He then traveled to the University of Texas Medical Branch in Galveston in the United States to pursue graduate studies under the guidance of Dr. William D. Willis, an internationally renowned neuroscientist in the field of pain research. Saab obtained his Ph.D. in 2001. His decision to join the department of neurology at Yale University as a postdoctoral fellow in 2001 soon put him on an exciting path toward better understanding the basic mechanisms of neuronal degeneration and reversal. He wrote this book partly while at Yale and the final stages while at Brown University and Rhode Island Hospital as an assistant professor-research at the department of surgery. Saab enjoys science and solving riddles, philosophy, and painting. Occasionally, you might also see him passing you on his road-racing bike at 20 miles per hour. He also enjoys working as a disc jockey at dance clubs.

# Picture Credits